Sclerotherapy in Dermatology

Sclerotherapy in Dermatology

Editors

Sacchidanand S DVD MD FRCP (Glasgow)
Dean/Director
Bangalore Medical College and Research Institute
Director of Medical Education
Government of Karnataka
Bengaluru, Karnataka, India

Nagesh TS MD DNB
Professor and Head
Sapthagiri Institute of Medical Sciences and
Research Center
Bengaluru, Karnataka, India

Foreword
Dinker Belle Rai MD FACS FRCS(c)

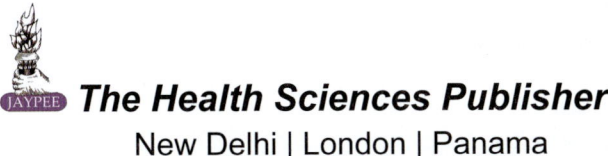

The Health Sciences Publisher
New Delhi | London | Panama

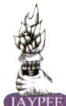 **Jaypee Brothers Medical Publishers (P) Ltd**

Headquarters

Jaypee Brothers Medical Publishers (P) Ltd
4838/24, Ansari Road, Daryaganj
New Delhi 110 002, India
Phone: +91-11-43574357
Fax: +91-11-43574314
Email: jaypee@jaypeebrothers.com

Overseas Offices

J.P. Medical Ltd
83 Victoria Street, London
SW1H 0HW (UK)
Phone: +44 20 3170 8910
Fax: +44 (0)20 3008 6180
Email: info@jpmedpub.com

Jaypee-Highlights Medical Publishers Inc
City of Knowledge, Bld. 235, 2nd Floor, Clayton
Panama City, Panama
Phone: +1 507-301-0496
Fax: +1 507-301-0499
Email: cservice@jphmedical.com

Jaypee Brothers Medical Publishers (P) Ltd
17/1-B Babar Road, Block-B, Shaymali
Mohammadpur, Dhaka-1207
Bangladesh
Mobile: +08801912003485
Email: jaypeedhaka@gmail.com

Jaypee Brothers Medical Publishers (P) Ltd
Bhotahity, Kathmandu, Nepal
Phone +977-9741283608
Email: kathmandu@jaypeebrothers.com

Website: www.jaypeebrothers.com
Website: www.jaypeedigital.com

© 2018, Jaypee Brothers Medical Publishers

The views and opinions expressed in this book are solely those of the original contributor(s)/author(s) and do not necessarily represent those of editor(s) of the book.

All rights reserved. No part of this publication may be reproduced, stored or transmitted in any form or by any means, electronic, mechanical, photocopying, recording or otherwise, without the prior permission in writing of the publishers.

All brand names and product names used in this book are trade names, service marks, trademarks or registered trademarks of their respective owners. The publisher is not associated with any product or vendor mentioned in this book.

Medical knowledge and practice change constantly. This book is designed to provide accurate, authoritative information about the subject matter in question. However, readers are advised to check the most current information available on procedures included and check information from the manufacturer of each product to be administered, to verify the recommended dose, formula, method and duration of administration, adverse effects and contraindications. It is the responsibility of the practitioner to take all appropriate safety precautions. Neither the publisher nor the author(s)/editor(s) assume any liability for any injury and/or damage to persons or property arising from or related to use of material in this book.

This book is sold on the understanding that the publisher is not engaged in providing professional medical services. If such advice or services are required, the services of a competent medical professional should be sought.

Every effort has been made where necessary to contact holders of copyright to obtain permission to reproduce copyright material. If any have been inadvertently overlooked, the publisher will be pleased to make the necessary arrangements at the first opportunity. The **CD/DVD-ROM** (if any) provided in the sealed envelope with this book is complimentary and free of cost. **Not meant for sale.**

Inquiries for bulk sales may be solicited at: jaypee@jaypeebrothers.com

Sclerotherapy in Dermatology

First Edition: **2018**
ISBN: 978-93-5270-206-0
Printed at: Samrat Offset Pvt. Ltd.

Contributors

Akhilesh A MD
Assistant Professor
Department of Dermatology
Sapthagiri Institute of
Medical Sciences and Research Center
Bengaluru, Karnataka, India

Savitha AS MD DNB FRGUHS
(Dermatosurgery)
Assistant Professor
Department of Dermatology
Sapthagiri Institute of
Medical Sciences and Research Center
Bengaluru, Karnataka, India

Nirmal B MD FRGUHS (Dermatosurgery)
Assistant Professor and Consultant
Department of Dermatology
Velammal Medical College Hospital
and Research Institute
Madurai, Tamil Nadu, India

Shashikumar BM MD
Associate Professor
Mandya Institute of Medical Sciences
Mandya, Karnataka, India

Shruthi C MD
Consultant Dermatologist
Bengaluru, Karnataka, India

Lakshmi DV DVD
Senior Resident
Bangalore Medical College and
Research Center
Bengaluru, Karnataka, India

Teresita S Ferrariz MD FPDS FPSCS
FPADSFI
Board of Directors, ISDS
Immediate Past President, PADSFI
Head on Accreditations
Dermatology Department
Centuria Medical Makati
Kalayaan Ave, Makati City, Philippines

Divya Gorur K MD FRGUHS
(Dermatosurgery)
Senior Resident
Bangalore Medical College and
Research Center
Bengaluru, Karnataka, India

Shilpa K MD FRGUHS
(Dermatosurgery)
Assistant Professor
Bangalore Medical College and
Research Center
Bengaluru, Karnataka, India

Dinker Belle Rai MD FACS FRCS(c)
Chairman
Department of Surgery
Interfaith Medical Center
Brooklyn, New York, USA
Visiting Associate Clinical Professor of
Surgery
SUNY Downstate Medical Center
Brooklyn
Visiting Professor of Surgery
Rajiv Gandhi University
Bengaluru, Karnataka, India

Late GR Ratnavel MD
Former Professor
Stanley Medical College
Chennai, Tamil Nadu, India

Sacchidanand S DVD MD FRCP
(Glasgow)
Dean/Director
Bangalore Medical College and
Research Institute
Director of Medical Education
Government of Karnataka
Bengaluru, Karnataka, India

Sujala S MD, FRGUHS (Dermatosurgery)
Consultant Dermatologist
Sujala Polyclinic
Bengaluru, Karnataka, India

Durganna T MS
Professor
Department of Surgery
Rajarajeswari Medical College and
Research Center
Bengaluru, Karnataka, India

Agnes E Thaebtharm MD
Fellow, Philippine Academy of
Dermatologic Surgery Foundation
Inc. Consultant at the Department of
Dermatology
Jose R Reyes Memorial Medical Center
Manila, Philippines

Nagesh TS MD DNB
Professor and Head
Sapthagiri Institute of
Medical Sciences and
Research Center
Bengaluru, Karnataka, India

Aniketh Venkataram MS MCH
(Plastic Surgery)
Consultant Plastic Surgeron
The Venkat Center for
Cosmetic and Plastic Surgery
Bengaluru, Karnataka, India

Foreword

At the outset, I am rejoicing a sense of accomplishment in writing this foreword on a book written on the system of the human body which happens to be the cause of the most common ailment in India and the rest of the world but hitherto is also the least attended area by the medical fraternity, i.e. diseases of the venous system. A field I passionately fell in love immediately after I finished my Vascular Surgery fellowship in 1979. No sooner I came in contact with a few like-minded physicians across the nation (USA) and we formed the first ever society for Venous diseases in US named the Phlebology Society of America. We began interchanging and propagating the new explorations. Venous field was in its primordial state in USA till then. This new movement soon kindled the interest of other physicians mainly from Surgery and Dermatology to establish new venous societies.

As a surgeon, my interest was not just cosmetic sclerotherapy, but the understanding of Chronic Venous Insufficiency Disease (CVID) in its entirety. CVID presents itself in its initial manifestation as spider veins, telangiectasia, reticular veins and superficial varicosity. In full blown form, presents large varicose veins, severe skin changes, swelling, intractable ulcers and inability of ambulation with pain on weight bearing. In the process of treatment, we revisited the old art of sclerotherapy. It was practiced by few physicians in 1920s in the US and eventually fell out of use because there was no scientific follow-up and interchange of the knowledge or meeting of the minds. No well organized written techniques of application. We re-explored and soon found that it is applicable both for cosmetic and therapeutic treatment of all kinds of superficial manifestation of CVID if done methodically. Found the possibility of replacing the age old surgery of ligating and stripping of the saphenous system for all kinds of CVID. This brought out a paradigm shift in understanding the underlying etiology of the disease, thereby changing the diagnostic modalities. Resulted in newer methods of nonsurgical treatment. It could be managed as outpatient office practice, affordable to common people and cost effective. At the same time more effectively, time saving for the patient and cosmetics to young ladies. Soon, we started giving workshops all over the world and became a new specialty by itself attracting mainly the attention of Dermatologists. Today, after practicing it for more than 35 years, I am pretty well convinced that sclerotherapy alone with minimal invasive procedure known as stab phlebectomy in selected patients can manage 95% of venous diseases on outpatient basis. Except 5%, which belong to deep venous system, may need surgical procedures.

In 2006, the prominent Dermatologists of Bengaluru, Dr Sacchidanand S, Dr SDN Gupta and Dr Venkatram Mysore invited me to give a Hands-on Workshop in Sclerotherapy, for the treatment of Varicose veins. This was done for Indian Association of Dermatologists, Venereologists and Leprologists during their conference held in Bengaluru. This opened a new door for the Indian dermatologists to take over the treatment of venous disease from the surgeons. Sclerotherapy was applied by them both as a cosmetic and therapeutic tool in as a single stroke.

I congratulate Dr Sacchidanand S and Dr Nagesh TS carrying the mantle and spreading this art of treatment across the nation to help millions of Indians suffering from venous problems. Especially, it is more important today as a large population of India suffering from venous ailments are left out of treatment and are helpless. Office sclerotherapy makes it very affordable, cost effective, simplified outpatient management. So, I am proud to be part of this movement as an Alumni of Bangalore Medical College. It gives me an incredible sense of fulfillment that I am a part of this great medical contribution to India.

I consider this a special honor for me to write the foreword to this book titled Sclerotherapy in Dermatology of which the chief editors are Dr Sachidanand S and Dr Nagesh TS. I admire their dedication and commitment. Let this be a useful manual guiding all beginners and as well as the rest of the practitioners who may be from other specialties and interested in this field including the surgeons.

"The secret of change is to focus all of your energy not on fighting the old, but on building the new"—**Socrates**.

Dinker Belle Rai MD FACS FRCS(c)
Chairman
Department of Surgery
Interfaith Medical Center
Brooklyn, New York, USA
Visiting Associate Clinical Professor of Surgery
SUNY Downstate Medical Center
Visiting Professor of surgery
Rajiv Gandhi University
Bengaluru, Karnataka, India

Preface

Dermatology is a branch of medicine which relies heavily on outpatient treatment and also managing several incapacitating diseases as inpatients. Dermatosurgery is evolving as a sub-specialty in itself and various newer surgical modalities of treatment have been added to the dermatosurgeons' armamentarium. Management of venous diseases from the dermatologist's point of view always involved treating the venous eczema and pigmentation. However, sclerotherapy has been widely being practiced by dermatologists in the west in the treatment of varicose veins and its manifestations.

Varicose veins and its skin manifestations is a very common problem presenting to the dermatology outpatient departments. Sclerotherapy done in the early stages is a very useful tool in the management of varicose veins and also to prevent the complications of varicose veins. However, not many books are available on this subject and also dermatologists are not practicing this procedure regularly.

Our book *Sclerotherapy in Dermatology* is an attempt to provide a simple and comprehensive guide to the practitioners about sclerotherapy. It includes the basics of venous anatomy and also the techniques of sclerotherapy. We would like more and more dermatologists to take up this simple and effective therapeutic procedure for the treatment of venous diseases. In this book, we also have given the extended indications of sclerotherapy in the management of cystic lesions and pyogenic granuloma. The target readers are postgraduate students, dermatologists, and surgeons. We hope to arouse interest in sclerotherapy among the dermatologists.

We hope that this book will provide the knowledge and confidence to clinicians and postgraduates to take up sclerotherapy in their practice.

Sacchidanand S
Nagesh TS

Acknowledgments

We would like to acknowledge the great help and support of Shri Jitendar P Vij (Group Chairman), Mr Ankit Vij (Group President), Ms Chetna Malhotra Vohra (Associate Director-Content Strategy), Ms Payal Bharti (Senior Manager) of M/s Jaypee Brothers Medical Publishers, New Delhi, India.

Contents

1. **Venous Anatomy** 1
   Aniketh Venkataram
   - Superficial Veins — 2
   - Deep Veins — 6
   - Perforating Veins — 7
   - Histology — 9
   - Related Nerves — 10

2. **Pathophysiology of Varicose Veins** 13
   Nirmal B
   - Physiology of Venous System of Lower Limbs — 14
   - Venous Pathophysiology — 15

3. **Skin Changes in Venous Insufficiency** 19
   Shashikumar BM, Savitha AS
   - Cosmetic Concerns — 20
   - Edema — 20
   - Corona Phlebectatica Paraplantaris (Ankle Flare) — 21
   - Superficial Thrombophlebitis — 21
   - Hemorrhage — 21
   - Pigmentation — 22
   - Pressure Erythema — 22
   - Eczema — 22
   - Lipodermatosclerosis — 23
   - Atrophie Blanche — 24
   - Ulceration — 24
   - Other Rare Complications — 26

4. **Evaluation of Varicose Veins** 29
   Shilpa K, Lakshmi DV, Divya Gorur K
   - History — 29
   - Bedside Tests — 31
   - Imaging Studies — 34

5. **Compression Therapy following Sclerotherapy** 41
   Late GR Ratnavel
   - Compression Therapy — 41
   - Types of Compression after Sclerotherapy — 43
   - What do Guidelines and Studies Say — 44
   - Time of Application of Compression Bandage — 44

6. **Sclerosing Solutions** 46
   Akhilesh A
   General Mechanism of Action of Sclerosants   46
   Detergents   47
   Osmotic Solutions   51
   Chemical Irritants   54
   Sequential Injections of Different Sclerosing Solutions   56
   Ideal Sclerosant   57

7. **Sclerotherapy for Varicose Veins** 63
   Nagesh TS, Sacchidanand S, Dinker Belle Rai
   History   63
   Indications of Sclerotherapy in Varicose Veins   64
   Contraindications   64
   Sclerosing Solutions   65
   Pre-procedure Assessment   66
   Sclerosant Concentrations   67
   Principles of Varicose Vein Sclerotherapy   67
   Patient Preparation   67
   Techniques   68

8. **Foam Sclerotherapy** 75
   Savitha AS, Sujala S
   History   75
   Methods of Foam Preparation   75
   Foam Stability   76
   Types of Foam   77
   Requirements   77
   Patient Position   78
   Sclerosing Agents   78
   Indications and Contraindications   78
   Procedure   79
   Postprocedure   80
   Complications   81
   Advantages of Foam Sclerotherapy   82

9. **Complications of Sclerotherapy** 85
   Teresita S Ferrariz, Agnes E Thaebtharm
   Prevention of Complications   85
   Complications   86
   Management of Complications   94
   Conflicts of Interest   98
   Acknowledgment   98

10. **Sclerotherapy for Cystic and Benign Vascular Lesions** 100
    Sacchidanand S, Nagesh TS, Shruthi C

Sebaceous Cyst/Epidermoid Cyst	100
Mucous Cyst and Ranula	101
Steatocystoma Multiplex	104
Lymphangioma Circumscriptum	104
Pyogenic Granuloma	106
Acknowledgments	109

11. **Surgical Treatment of Varicose Veins** 111
    Durganna T

History	111
Saphenofemoral Ligation and Long Saphenous Stripping	112
Saphenopopliteal Junction Ligation and Lesser Saphenous Stripping	114
Perforator Ligation	115
Phlebectomies	116
Conservative Venous Ligation	117
Postoperative Instructions	118
Complications of Standard Varicose Vein Surgery	118
Minimal Invasive Methods	118
Radiofrequency Ablation	120
Recurrent Varicose Veins	120
Comparison of Interventions	121

Index   123

CHAPTER 1

Venous Anatomy

Aniketh Venkataram

INTRODUCTION

Knowledge of venous anatomy is essential for diagnosis and treatment of venous disorders of the lower limb. Venous anatomy was largely ignored in earlier anatomy textbooks, and its importance underappreciated. However, with increase in interest in venous disease and advent of newer imaging methods, much information has been gathered in this field. The unique anatomy in the lower limbs enables veins to act both as a reservoir of excess blood as well as a conduit for the return of blood to the heart.

Knowledge of fascial anatomy of the lower limb is essential to understand the venous anatomy. The veins of the lower limb can be divided into superficial and deep veins, with the deep muscle fascia separating the two. The superficial compartment consists of all tissue between the skin and the deep muscle fascia, and the deep compartment consists of all the tissue between the fascia and the bones. The saphenous compartment is a component of the superficial compartment enclosed between the saphenous fascia and the deep muscle fascia (Fig. 1.1). Communicating veins connect veins within the same compartment whereas perforator veins connect superficial and deep veins.[1] With this background, we shall review the venous anatomy under the following headings: (1) superficial veins, (2) deep veins and (3) perforating veins.

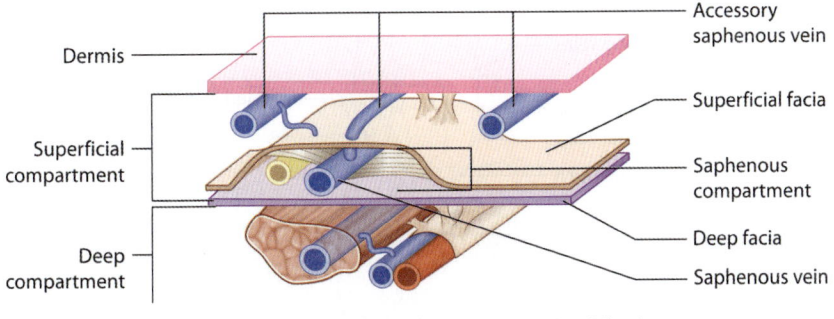

Fig. 1.1: Superficial fascial compartments of the leg.

SUPERFICIAL VEINS

In the skin, capillaries drain into a subpapillary venous plexus which drains into a deeper reticular plexus at the dermal subcutaneous junction. Vertically oriented veins connect the reticular plexus to the superficial veins.

Few veins in the body are more variable than the superficial veins of the lower limb. They begin in the foot with the dorsal and plantar venous plexuses. On the dorsum of the foot, small superficial veins form the dorsal venous arch at the level of the proximal end of the metatarsals. This forms the great and small saphenous veins (SSVs) at its medial and lateral ends respectively (Fig. 1.2).[2]

Great Saphenous Vein

This begins at the medial end of the dorsal venous arch and ascends 2.5–3 cm anterior to the medial malleolus. It crosses the distal third of the medial surface of the tibia obliquely to its medial border. It ascends a little behind the medial border and crosses the knee posteromedial to the medial tibial and femoral condyles. It runs on the medial side of the thigh and enters the fossa ovalis 3 cm below and lateral to the pubic tubercle. At this point, it drains into the femoral vein at the saphenofemoral junction (SFJ). The surface anatomy is marked from this point to the adductor tubercle of the femur. The SFJ however is highly variable and the surface marking is not reliable (Fig. 1.3).[3]

Tributaries

In the calf, the great saphenous vein (GSV) has two main tributaries, the anterior and posterior arch veins. The posterior arch vein, also called Leonardo's vein (first depicted in Da Vinci's drawing) drains a fine network below the

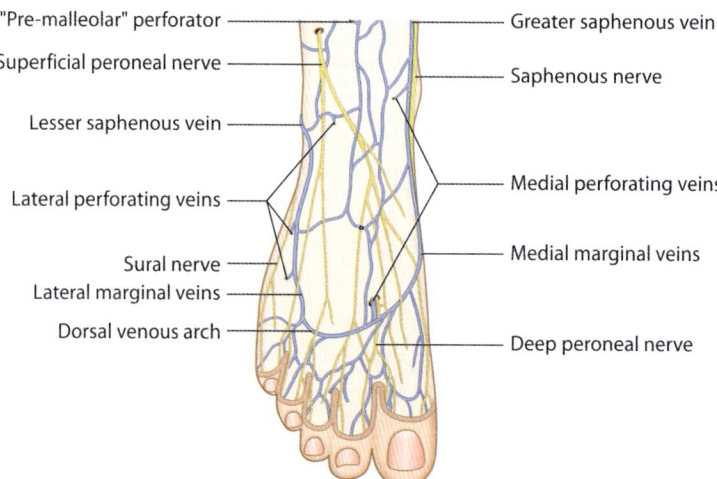

Fig. 1.2: Veins of the foot.

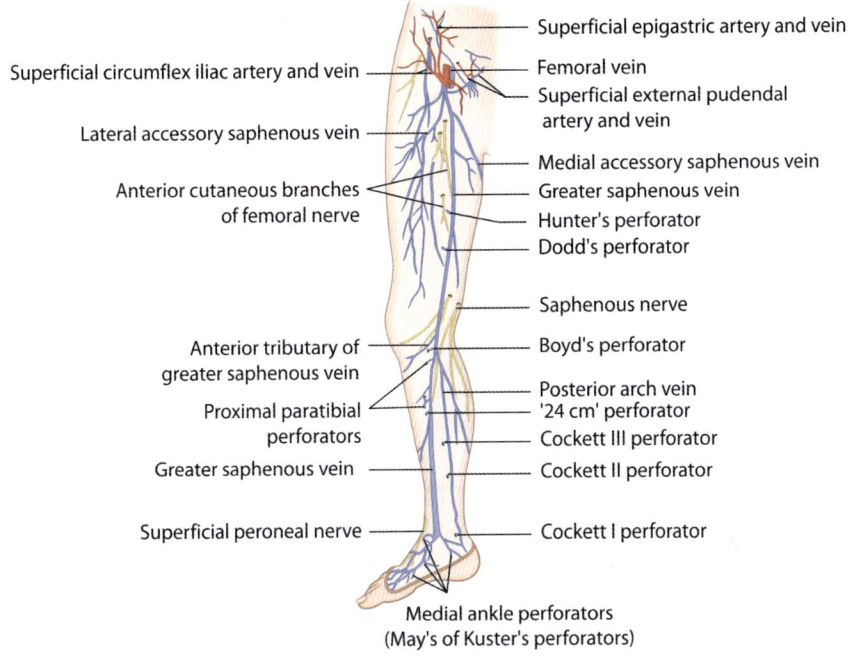

Fig. 1.3: Great saphenous vein.

medial ankle, ascends on medial aspect of the lower half of the leg and joins the GSV just distal to the knee. The Cockett's perforators connect the posterior arch vein to the posterior tibial veins as shall be seen later. There are several other variable, unnamed communications with the SSV.

In the thigh, the GSV receives the lateral and medial accessory saphenous veins. The lateral is more consistent and drains the anterolateral aspect of the thigh. The medial vein is present in 8–20% of cases, and drains the posterior aspect of the thigh. Both veins may be mistaken for the GSV. A recent study has classified the GSV as medial dominant, lateral dominant or equal based on the drainage of these accessory saphenous veins.[4]

Saphenofemoral Junction

Just before the SFJ, the GSV receives the superficial external pudendal, superficial external iliac, and the superficial inferior epigastric veins. A little more distally is the drainage of the medial and lateral accessory saphenous veins. Various attempts have been made to classify the confluence of veins at the SFJ, but none are reliable due to the high variability of this confluence. Most commonly what has been described is a venous star, as shown in Figure 1.4, involving the five main tributaries. But there can be any number of patterns of the tributaries draining into each other, or separately into the femoral vein.[5]

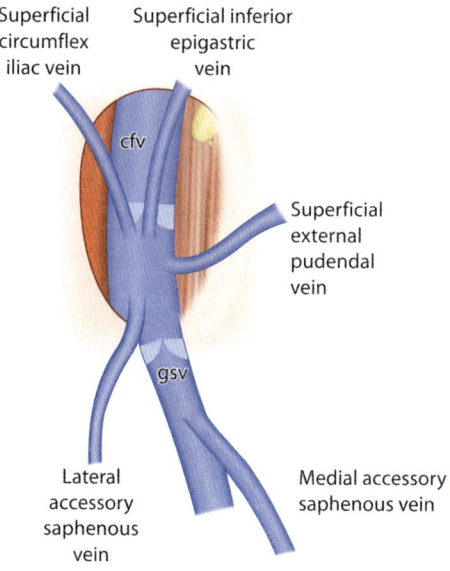

Fig. 1.4: Saphenofemoral junction.

Small Saphenous Vein

It begins on the lateral aspect of the dorsal venous arch, runs behind the lateral malleolus and ascends lateral to the Achilles tendon. In the upper third of the leg, it pierces the deep fascia between the two heads of the gastrocnemius and empties into the popliteal vein in the proximal popliteal fossa at the saphenopopliteal junction (SPJ). In a third of patients, it empties high into the femoral vein or the GSV. Its surface marking is from a point midway between the bottom of the lateral malleolus and the tendoachilles to the midpoint of the knee joint line.[2]

Tributaries

There are several communicating branches between the SSV and the GSV. In 15% of patients, there is a large communicating vein named after Giacomini which connects the proximal part of the SSV to the GSV. There are other small communications between the saphenous veins around the knee (Fig. 1.5).[6]

Saphenopopliteal Junction

The termination of the SPJ is highly variable. A short time ago, a universally accepted classification for the SPJ was established. Type A is the classical SPJ. Type B is when the SSV empties into the SPJ with another cranial extension into the GSV or SFJ. Type C is when there is no SPJ, but the vein empties higher up (Fig. 1.6).[7]

Venous Anatomy

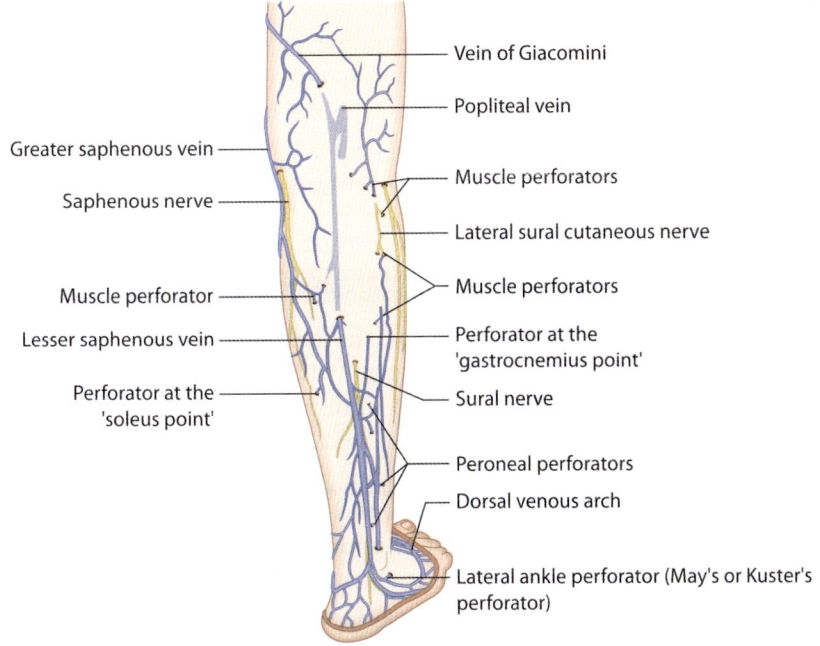

Fig. 1.5: Small saphenous vein.

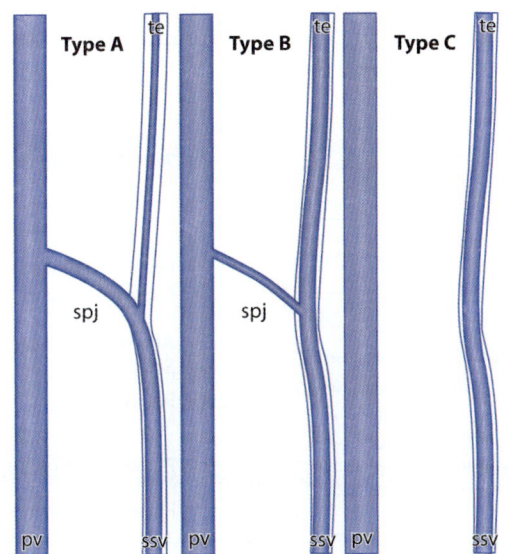

Fig. 1.6: Saphenopopliteal junction.

Valves

In the superficial veins, bicuspid valves exist which direct blood flow towards the heart. There are larger valves at termination of venous trunks with strong cusps and sinusoidal dilatation of the vein wall. The GSV usually has 6–14 valves, which are more numerous in the leg than the thigh. One valve called the preterminal valve is present as it pierces the cribriform fascia. The terminal valve is present at its junction with the femoral vein. The SSV has 4–13 valves which are more closely spaced, with the highest valve at the termination of the SSV. Valves in communicating tributaries direct blood from the SSV to the GSV.[8]

DEEP VEINS

The deep plantar arch collects blood from the toes and metatarsum. This then forms the medial and lateral plantar veins, which form the posterior tibial vein behind the medial ankle. The major dorsal deep veins (dorsalis pedis) form the anterior tibial veins.[9]

In the calf, these veins run in pairs. The posterior tibial veins drain the muscles of the posterior compartments and run between the flexor digitorum longus and the tibialis posterior. They drain the GSV and posterior arch veins via perforators. They then pierce the soleus and continue as the popliteal vein.

The anterior tibial veins drain the muscles of the anterior compartment. The peroneal veins form in the lower third of the leg below the flexor hallucis longus. They receive peroneal perforators as well as veins form the soleus muscle. The anterior tibial and peroneal veins form the tibioperoneal trunk which drains into the popliteal vein (Fig. 1.7).[2]

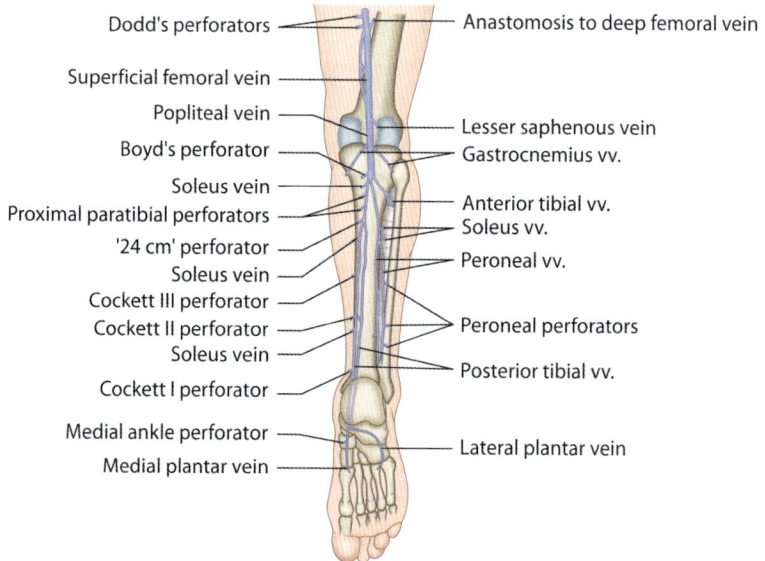

Fig. 1.7: Deep veins of the lower limb.

In the popliteal fossa, the vein is deep to the artery, but it then ascends and crosses the artery from medial to lateral in a superficial position. In the adductor canal, it becomes the superficial femoral vein which drains the medial side of the thigh and is connected by perforators to the GSV. The profunda femoris vein drains the lateral thigh and receives perforators form the lateral accessory saphenous vein. About 9 cm below the inguinal ligament, it joins the femoral vein to form the common femoral vein, which receives the GSV at the SFJ. It also receives the medial and lateral circumflex femoral veins. It lies medial to the artery at the inguinal canal and continues as the external iliac vein.[8]

The deep veins of the foot and distal calf have many valves at 2 cm intervals. The thigh deep veins have very few valves. There is one constant valve at the junction of the superficial femoral and profunda femoris.

Venous Sinuses of Calf Muscles

These are thin walled venous reservoirs in the calf muscles, which contract during ambulation. They act as a peripheral muscle pump to aid in venous return against gravity. The soleus is rich with sinuses while the gastrocnemius has few. These sinuses are filled by superficial veins via indirect perforators and via muscular veins. They drain into deep veins via soleus and gastrocnemius veins. The sinuses themselves have no valves, but their draining veins do. These valves are vital for the efficiency of the peripheral muscle pump (Fig. 1.8).[10]

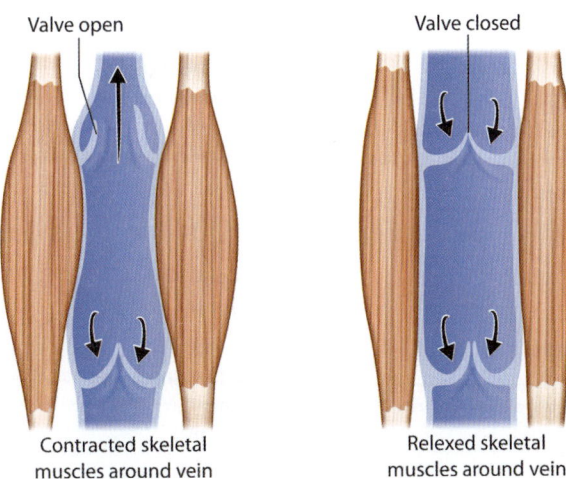

Fig. 1.8: Peripheral calf muscle pump.

PERFORATING VEINS

Perforating veins are either direct in which case they drain into deep veins, or indirect where they drain into deep veins via calf muscle sinuses. Small communicating branches often connect perforators to one another. There perforators usually have one to three valves which direct blood flow from superficial to deep. The number of perforating veins has been variably reported in various studies, with as many as 150 been reported.

Of these, there are four groups of significant perforators: foot, medial calf, lateral calf and thigh. These perforators were initially named after their finders (e.g., Boyd, Cockett). However, in 2001, the International Union of Angiology decided on a standard nomenclature for these to aid in information exchange and standardization.[11] The direct perforators usually have a reliable anatomy while the indirect perforators are unpredictably distributed (Table 1.1).

Table 1.1: Perforator nomenclature.

Foot perforators	Dorsal foot PV or intercapitular veins Medial foot PV Lateral foot PV Plantar foot PV
Ankle perforators	Anterior ankle PV Lateral ankle PV
Leg perforator	Medial leg PV • Paratibial PV • Posterior tibial PV (Cockett PV) Anterior leg PV Lateral leg PV Posterior leg PV Medial gastrocnemius PV Lateral gastrocnemius PV Intergemellar PV Para-Achillean PV
Knee perforators	Medial knee PV Suprapatellar PV Lateral knee PV Infrapatellar PV Popliteal fossa PV
Thigh perforators	Medial thigh PV • PV of the femoral canal • Inguinal PV Anterior thigh PV Lateral thigh PV Posterior thigh PV • Posteromedial • Sciatic PV • Posterolateral Pudendal PV

PV: Perforating veins.

Foot Perforators

The foot usually has around 10 perforators. One large one in the first web space connects the superficial venous arch to the dorsalis pedis. On the medial aspect, perforators connect the GSV to the dorsalis pedis. On the lateral aspect, perforators connect the SSV to the lateral plantar deep vein. The ankle perforators were previously named after May and Kuster.[9]

Medial Calf Perforators

The medial calf perforators are clinically the most significant. They were formerly named after Cockett into three groups; Cockett I (behind malleolus), Cockett II (7-9 cm from tip of medial malleolus) and Cockett III (10-12 cm from malleolus). These are all located 2-4 cm from the medial edge of the tibia and average 7-8 in number. These connect the GSV and posterior arch vein with the posterior tibial veins. In the upper half of the leg, perforators are located more closely to the tibia and are called paratibial perforators. They are usually seen in three groups; at distances of 18-22, 23-27 and 28-32 cm from the medial malleolus. The 18-22 cm group was also called the 24 cm perforator due to its distance from the sole. These perforators drain the GSV, and its tributaries into the posterior tibial veins. Just distal to the knee, there is another consistent set of perforators formerly called Boyd's perforators which connect the GSV to the popliteal veins.[12]

Lateral Calf Perforators

On the lateral calf, the peroneal perforators connect the SSV to the peroneal vein. Named ones include the Bassi's perforator at 5-7 cm from lateral malleolus and the 12 cm perforator at 12-14 cm from the lateral malleolus. More proximally, perforators are usually indirect. On the anterior calf, the perforators of note include the premalleolar and midcrural ones which drain GSV into anterior tibial vein.[13]

Thigh Perforators

In the thigh, direct perforators are less frequent. They include the Dodd's and Hunterian perforators to the popliteal and superficial femoral respectively. Several indirect perforators to the muscular veins exist (Fig. 1.9).[14]

HISTOLOGY

The vein wall is made up of three layers; the intima, media and adventitia. The intima consists of a single layer of endothelial cells lying on connective tissue. Valves are made up of connective tissue with intima on both sides. The media is made up of smooth muscle cells and connective tissue. Larger veins

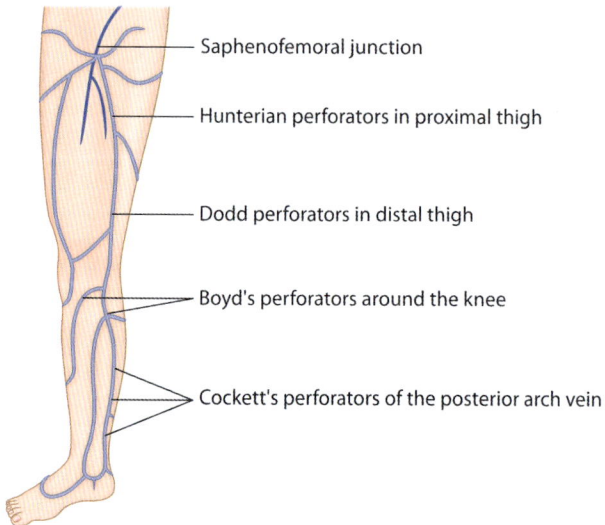

Fig. 1.9: Major perforator veins of the lower limb.

have more smooth muscle and are resistant to varicosity. Smaller tributaries have less muscle and are more prone for varicosity. The adventitia is poorly demarcated and contains vessels, nerves and lymphatics.[15]

Previously, it was thought that valves are absent in smaller veins, but recent studies have proven otherwise. Microvascular valves have been demonstrates in collecting venules and smaller caliber veins up to 1,000 microns. The functional significance of this finding is as yet incompletely understood.[16]

RELATED NERVES

Saphenous Nerve

The saphenous nerve descends with the superficial femoral artery, deep to the sartorius. It gives an infrapatellar branch to supply the skin medial to the knee. The main nerve pierces the fascia lata above the knee and becomes superficial between the gracilis and sartorius, at which point it is deep and posterior to the GSV. Below this point, it becomes more superficial and anterior, and is eventually juxtaposed with the GSV, around 2-3 cm below and medial to the tibial tuberosity. The nerve then travels close to the GSV, which makes vein removal almost impossible without nerve injury. Eventually it terminates by supply skin over medial leg and foot.

Sural Nerve

This nerve arises from the tibial nerve in the popliteal fossa, descends in the posterior leg to the back of the lateral malleolus. It lies on the lateral head of the gastrocnemius and then lies in the groove between the two heads, lateral to the SSV. It usually pierces the deep fascia with the SSV and then courses close to the SSV. It terminates by supplying the skin over posterior half and lateral foot.[17]

CONCLUSION

In conclusion, venous anatomy of the lower limb is one of the most variable and unpredictable in the entire body. A thorough knowledge of the most common patterns enable us to identify variations when they arise; thereby ensuring adequate identification and treatment of various venous disorders.

REFERENCES

1. May R. Nomenclature of the surgically most important connecting veins. In: May R, Partsch H, Staubesand J (Eds). Perforating Veins. Baltimore: Urban & Schwartzenberg; 1981. pp. 13-8.
2. Mozes G, Carmichael SW, Gloviczi P. Development and anatomy of the venous system. In: Gloviczki P (Ed). Handbook of Venous Disorders (2nd edition). London (UK): Arnold Publishers; 2001. pp. 11-24.
3. Caggiati A, Bergan JJ. The Saphenous vein: derivation of its name and its relevant anatomy. J Vasc Surg. 2002;35(1):172-5.
4. Shah DM, Chang BB, Leopold PW, et al. The anatomy of the greater saphenous venous system. J Vasc Surg. 1986;3(2):273-83.
5. Mühlberger D, Morandini L, Brenner E. Venous valves and major superficial tributary veins near the saphenofemoral junction. J Vasc Surg. 2009;49(6):1562-9.
6. Delis KT, Knaggs AL, Khodabakhsh P. Prevalence, anatomic patterns, valvular competence, and clinical significance of the Giacomini vein. J Vasc Surg. 2004; 40(6):1174-83.
7. Schweighofer G, Mühlberger D, Brenner E. The anatomy of the small saphenous vein: fascial and neural relations, saphenofemoral junction, and valves. J Vasc Surg. 2010;51(4):982-9.
8. Dodd H, Cockett FB. Surgical anatomy of the veins of the lower limb. In: Dodd H, Cockett FB (Eds). The Pathology and Surgery of the Veins of the Lower Limb. London: E&S Livingstone; 1996. pp. 28-64.
9. Kuster G, Lofgren EP, Hollinshead WH. Anatomy of the veins of the foot. Surg Gynecol Obstet. 1968;127(4): 817-23.
10. Ludbrook J. The musculovenous pumps of the human lower limb. Am Heart J. 1966;71(5):635-41.
11. Caggiati A, Bergan JJ, Gloviczki P, et al. International Interdisciplinary Consensus Committee on Venous Anatomical Terminology. Nomenclature of the veins of the lower limb: extensions, refinements, and clinical application. J Vasc Surg. 2005;41(4):719-24.
12. Mozes G, Gloviczki P, Menawat SS, et al. Surgical anatomy for endoscopic subfascial division of perforating veins. J Vasc Surg. 1996;24(5):800-8.
13. Thomson H. The surgical anatomy of the superficial and perforating veins of the lower limb. Ann R Coll Surg Engl. 1979;61(3):198-205.
14. Sherman RS. Varicose veins: anatomic findings and an operative procedure based upon them. Ann Surg. 1944;120(5):722-84.

15. Parum DV. Histochemistry and immunohistochemistry of vascular disease. In: Stehbens WE, Lie JT (Eds). Vascular Pathology. London: Chapman & Hall; 1995. pp. 313-27.
16. Caggiati A, Phillips M, Lametschwandtner A, et al. Valves in small veins and venules. Eur J Vasc Endovasc Surg. 2006;32(4):447-52.
17. Sam RC, Silverman SH, Bradbury AW. Nerve injuries and varicose vein surgery. Eur J Vasc Endovasc Surg. 2004;27(2):113-20.

CHAPTER 2

Pathophysiology of Varicose Veins

Nirmal B

INTRODUCTION

Venous diseases of the lower limbs are extremely complex due to wide variability of veins on the surface of the skin. It is important to understand the normal anatomy and physiology of veins of lower limbs with regard to management of pathology of leg veins. Venous hypertension leads to alterations in vein wall, valve incompetence and chronic venous insufficiency.

Anatomy of Venous System of Lower Limbs

The venous system of lower limbs is formed by:
- Superficial compartment
- Deep compartment
- Perforating veins

The superficial compartment (Fig. 2.1) comprises of three tributaries namely, greater saphenous vein (GSV), short saphenous vein (SSV) and lateral subdermic venous system (LSVS) of Albanese. It carries only 10% of the venous blood flow from the lower limb which drains eventually at the saphenofemoral

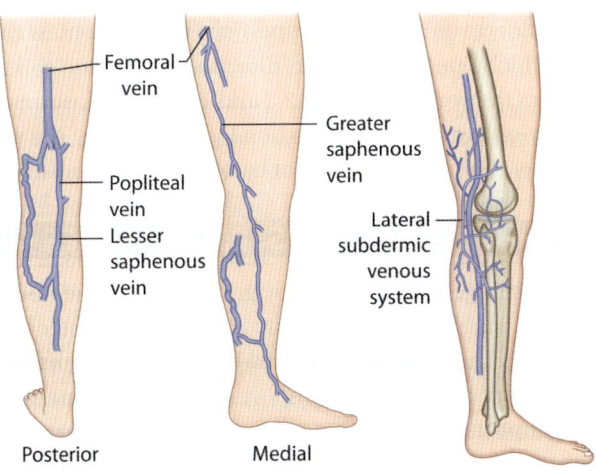

Fig. 2.1: Anatomy of the superficial compartment of venous system of the leg.

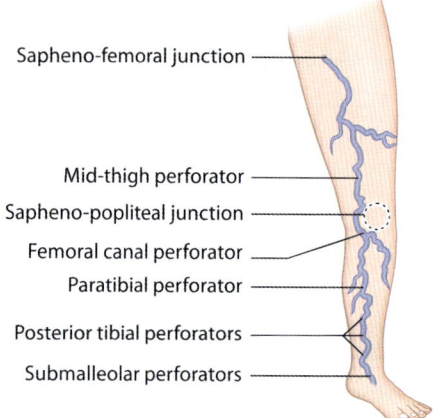

Fig. 2.2: Perforators of lower limbs.

Table 2.1: Old and new terminologies of perforators.	
Old terminology	**New terminology**
Hunterian	Mid-thigh perforator
Dodd	Femoral canal perforator
Boyd	Paratibial perforator
Crockett	Posterior tibial perforator
May	Ankle perforator

junction (SFJ). Intersaphenous vein of Giacomini located in the posteromedial aspect of leg connects GSV to SSV.

The deep venous system includes the femoral, popliteal, anterior tibial, posterior tibial and peroneal veins. It carries about 90% of venous return from the lower limbs. The flow of blood is from superficial to deep venous compartment through valves which open only in that direction. When the calf muscle contracts, the valves of the perforators (Fig. 2.2 and Table 2.1) close and blood flows only in one direction against gravity proximally to the heart. The venous valves in the deep venous compartment prevent backflow during muscle relaxation.[1]

PHYSIOLOGY OF VENOUS SYSTEM OF LOWER LIMBS

Venous pressure is largely determined by gravity. When the body is horizontal, venous pressure in the lower extremity is equal to that of lower abdomen. As the body becomes upright, the pressure in the lower limbs increases dramatically. Integrity of calf muscle pump, venous compartments, perforators and valves are important to counter the hydrostatic pressure due to gravity. Venous tone is the normal venous wall contraction in response to filling up with venous blood. Tone is important to maintain the venous pressure within

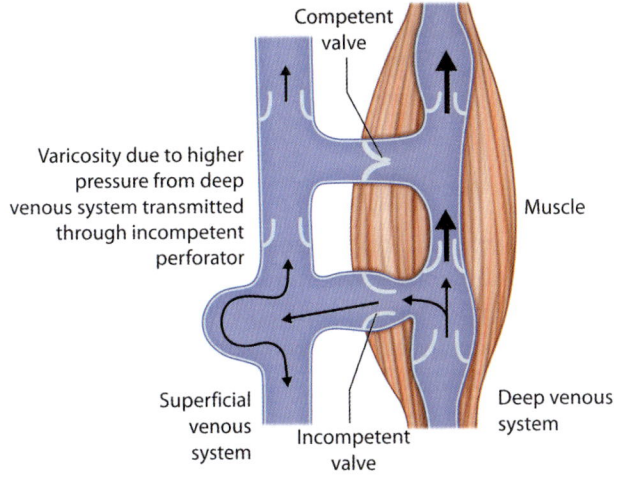

Fig. 2.3: Venous physiology of lower limbs.

normal limits. Valve closes when the vertical flow pressure exceeds the proximally directed jet flow pressure (Fig. 2.3).[2]

In normal individuals, venous pressure in the superficial compartment falls when the calf muscle pump contracts. As venous insufficiency develops, the high pressure of the deep compartment gets transferred to the superficial compartment and the venous pressure in the superficial compartment increases. A sustained elevation of ambulatory venous pressure in the superficial compartment leads to edema, hyperpigmentation, stasis dermatitis, varicose veins, venous ulcers and lipodermatosclerosis.[3]

VENOUS PATHOPHYSIOLOGY

The lower limb pathophysiological changes can be grouped under:
- Primary venous insufficiency—telangiectasia, reticular veins, varicose veins
- Chronic venous insufficiency—hyperpigmentation, ulcers, scarring, lipodermatosclerosis[4]

Primary Venous Insufficiency

The risk factors of primary venous insufficiency include:[5]
- *Age*: The prevalence increases with age due to compounding factors including calf muscle weakness and decrease in matrix proteins.
- *Sex*: Most studies show that varicose veins are commoner in women attributing also that women recognize them early and report.
- *Family history*: Varicose veins are 20 times more common in patients with a positive family history.
- *Genetics*: Though no specific gene mutation has been identified specific for varicose veins, few genetic disorders have been found associated with

Table 2.2: Vessel size and definition.		
Vessel	**Size**	**Synonyms**
Telangiectasia	<1 mm	Spider veins, thread veins
Reticular veins	1–3 mm	Blue veins, venulectasia
Varicose veins	>3 mm	Varices, varicosities

varicose veins namely, Klippel–Trenaunay syndrome, *FOXC2* mutation in lymphedema–distichiasis syndrome, *COL3A1* gene in Ehlers–Danlos syndrome, von Hippel–Lindau gene and *NOTCH3* mutation in cerebral autosomal dominant arteriopathy with subcortical infarcts and leukoencephalopathy (CADASIL).

- *Pregnancy*: Raised intra-abdominal pressure and increased levels of hormone-induced vasodilation such as relaxin, estrogen and progesterone increases the prevalence in pregnancy.
- *Others*: Obesity, cigarette smoking, estrogen therapy, decreased mobility, hypertension and diabetes are other risk factors of varicose veins.

The causes of primary venous insufficiency include:[6]

- Obstruction to venous return—thrombosis, radiation fibrosis
- Elevation of right atrial pressure—pulmonary hypertension, heart failure
- Failure of calf muscle pump—impairment of leg muscle function or joint mobility
- Failure of valves in the perforating veins
- Failure of valves in the deep venous system

Most common cause of valvular failure is thrombosis. Valve cusp is usually the nidus for thrombus. When plasmin lyses thrombus, the valve function is also lost. Venous system dysfunction either due to injury to venous walls or valves causes veins to elongate and dilate resulting in telangiectasia, reticular veins and varicose veins (Table 2.2). Recent evidence suggests vessel wall changes precede valve dysfunction.[7]

Chronic Venous Insufficiency

Venous dilatation and valve dysfunction resulting in venous microcirculation changes leads to interference with the nutrition of skin. A multicausal model of chronic venous insufficiency has been proposed by the University Hospital of Maastricht, Netherlands.[8] Raised pressure in the venular side of capillaries results in widening of interendothelial spaces. Plasma diffuses through these spaces leading to edema. Later, larger molecules, such as fibrinogen, diffuse and get converted into fibrin forming a cuff around the vessel wall. The fibrin cuff acts as a diffusion barrier for oxygen and growth factors. The widened capillaries have low flow velocity leading to capillary stasis. The white blood cellss in the veins form thrombi and block circulation (Fig. 2.4).

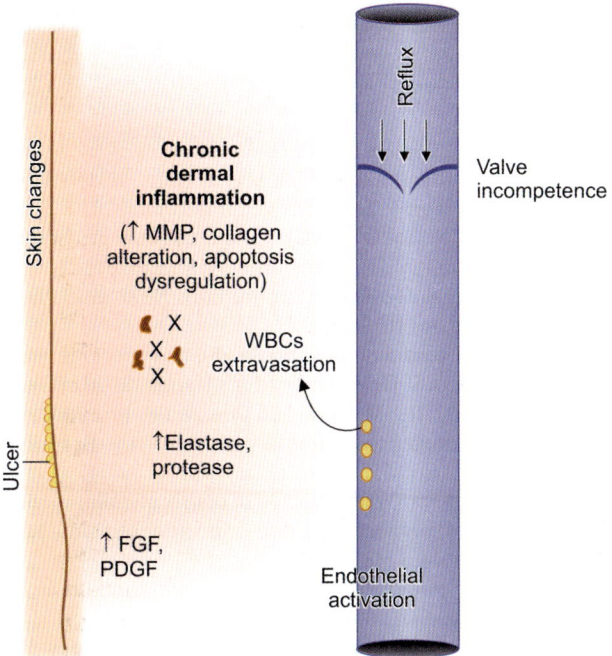

Fig. 2.4: Summary of the mechanisms that may contribute to varicose vein formation. ECM: Extracellular matrix; TIMP: Tissue inhibitor of metalloproteinase; SMC: Smooth muscle cell.

The various microvascular changes leading to chronic venous insufficiency includes:[9]

- *Extracellular matrix degradation:* The balance between matrix metalloproteinases (MMPs) and tissue inhibitors of metalloproteinases (TIMPs) maintains the homeostasis of extracellular matrix (ECM). Overexpression of *MMP-2* and *MMP-9* results in venous wall relaxation. Activity of *MMP-9* is a sensitive marker of venous stasis.[10]
- *Endothelial activation:* Injured endothelial cells release inflammatory mediators and growth factors (basic fibroblast growth factor and platelet-derived growth factor). These factors induce smooth muscle migration and dedifferentiation. Activated leucocytes may also release large amounts of superoxide anions and proteases that are able to degrade the ECM.
- *Smooth muscle dedifferentiation:* Smooth muscle cells (SMCs) in varicose veins shifts from contractile phenotype to proliferative phenotype. A decrease in actin cytoskeleton and fibronectin results in decreased contractility of varicose veins. SMCs and fibroblasts from patients with varicose veins synthesize significantly greater amounts of collagen I than collagen III.
- *Smooth muscle apoptosis dysregulation:* The expression of *bax* and *caspase 9* is decreased significantly in SMCs of varicose veins resulting in dysregulation of intrinsic apoptotic pathway.

REFERENCES

1. Bergan JJ, Pascarella L, Bunke N. Venous Anatomy, Physiology and Pathophysiology. In: Alam M, Silapunt S (Eds). Treatment of Leg Veins (2nd edition). Saunders: Elsevier; 2011. pp. 1-9.
2. Mortimer PS, Burnand KG, Neumann HAM. Diseases of the veins and arteries: Leg ucers. In: Burns T, Breathnach S, Cox N, et al. (Eds). Textbook of Dermatology (8th edition). West Sussex: Wiley-Blackwell Publishers; 2010. pp. 25-8.
3. Burton CS, Burkhart CN, Goldsmith LA. Cutaneous changes in venous and lymphatic insufficiency. In: Wolff K, Goldsmith LA, Katz SI, et al. (Eds). Fitzpatrick's Dermatology in General Medicine (7th edition). New York: The McGraw-Hill Companies Inc; 2008. pp. 1679-81.
4. Weiss RA, Weiss MA. Treatment for varicose and telangiectatic veins. In: Wolff K, Goldsmith LA, Katz SI, et al. (Eds). Fitzpatrick's Dermatology in General Medicine (7th edition). New York: The McGraw-Hill Companies Inc; 2008. pp. 2349-52.
5. Lim CS, Davies AH. Pathogenesis of primary varicose veins. Br J Surg. 2009; 96(11): 1231-42.
6. Chang JW, Maeng YH, Kim SW. Expression of matrix metalloproteinase-2 and -13 and tissue inhibitor of metalloproteinase-4 in varicose veins. Korean J Thorac Cardiovasc Surg. 2011;44(6):387-91.
7. Naoum JJ, Hunter GC. Pathogenesis of varicose veins and implications for clinical management. Vascular. 2007;15(5):242-9.
8. Bergan JJ. A unifying concept of primary venous insufficiency. Dermatol Surg. 1998;24(4):425-8.
9. Lim CS, Gohel MS, Shepherd AC, et al. Venous hypoxia: a poorly studied etiological factor of varicose veins. J Vasc Res. 2011;48(3):185-94.
10. Kucukguven A, Khalil RA. Matrix metalloproteinases as potential targets in the venous dilation associated with varicose veins. Curr Drug Targets. 2013; 14(3):287-324.

CHAPTER 3

Skin Changes in Venous Insufficiency

Shashikumar BM, Savitha AS

INTRODUCTION

Venous insufficiency is one of the commonest causes for eczema and pigment changes over the lower limbs. It can occur due to number of reasons. Most common are the occupations which involve standing for prolonged period of time. The vein valves and walls are affected by the progesterone levels cyclical changes in females. During pregnancy when the blood volume increases and venous return is hindered by gravid uterus, these venous changes are exacerbated. The atrophy of vessel wall smooth muscle which occur with age, makes the vein susceptible to dialation.[1]

Varicose veins are often symptomatic in addition to being unsightly. A German study found symptoms in 98% of patients with 'clinically relevant' venous alterations. A significant proportion of patients complain of lower limb symptoms, which they attribute to varicose veins. They are heaviness, swelling, aching, restless legs, itching, tingling and discoloration. Uncomplicated varicose veins are rarely painful. Pain may be related to pressure on the network of somatic nerve fibers in the subcutaneous tissues adjacent to the affected vein.[2] The severity of symptoms depends on the extent of high back pressure.

Patients with varicose veins present in one of the three categories: cosmetic, symptomatic or with one of the complications of venous disease (Table 3.1). The assessment of patients in the cosmetic group is relatively simple as the problem can be clearly seen.[3]

Table 3.1: Varicose vein presentation.

Group 1 Cosmetic only	Group 2 Symptomatic	Group 3 Complications
Venous telangiectasia Visible varicose veins	Aching on dependency or before periods Heaviness in the legs Itching Cramps Swelling Restless legs Tenderness Paresthesia	Bleeding from trauma Superficial phlebitis Ankle venous flare Atrophie blanche Venous eczema Lipodermatosclerosis +/− inflammatory component Venous ulcers

The commonest symptom is tired and aching sensation in the affected lower limb particularly in the calf at the end of the day. Easy fatigability and a heavy feeling after prolonged standing are present. Some patients suffer from cramp shortly after retiring to bed, which is usually due to sudden change in the caliber of communicating veins, which stimulates the muscles through which they pass. Pain may also be bursting or severe in nature and may be particularly localized to the site of incompetent perforating veins, and bursting pain during walking indicates deep vein deficiency.[4]

COSMETIC CONCERNS

Many patients seek treatment due to the unsightly appearance of varicose veins (Fig. 3.1). This is not only confined just to tortuous large veins but also to telangiectasia and reticular veins (Fig. 3.2). Telangiectasias have a variety of patterns like stellate, sunburst, and arborizing. Rarely, they may become so extensive as to give a blue-purplish discoloration to the entire leg. As women are more concerned with the appearance of the legs, there is a driving demand for treatment of varicose veins.[5]

EDEMA

In uncomplicated varicose veins, there will be mild ankle edema which becomes more prominent toward the end of the day. The edema is more severe and persistent in deep system insufficiency.[1]

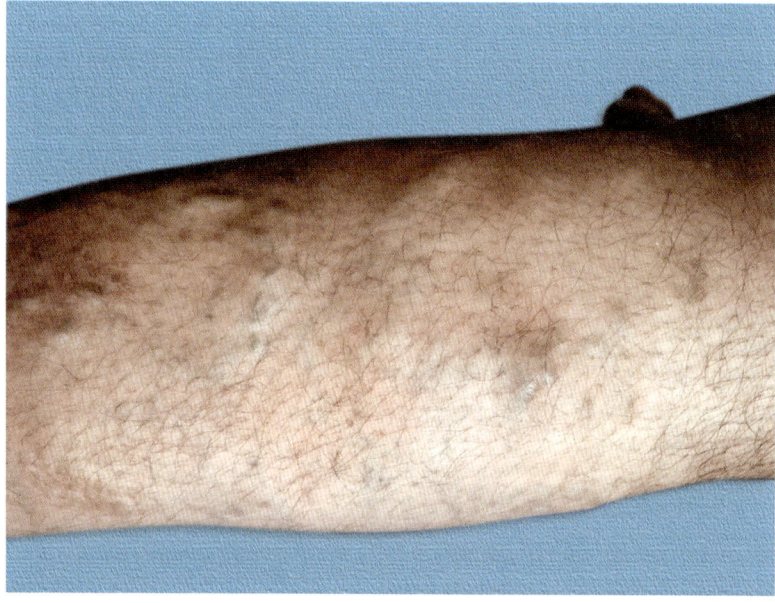

Fig. 3.1: Varicose veins.

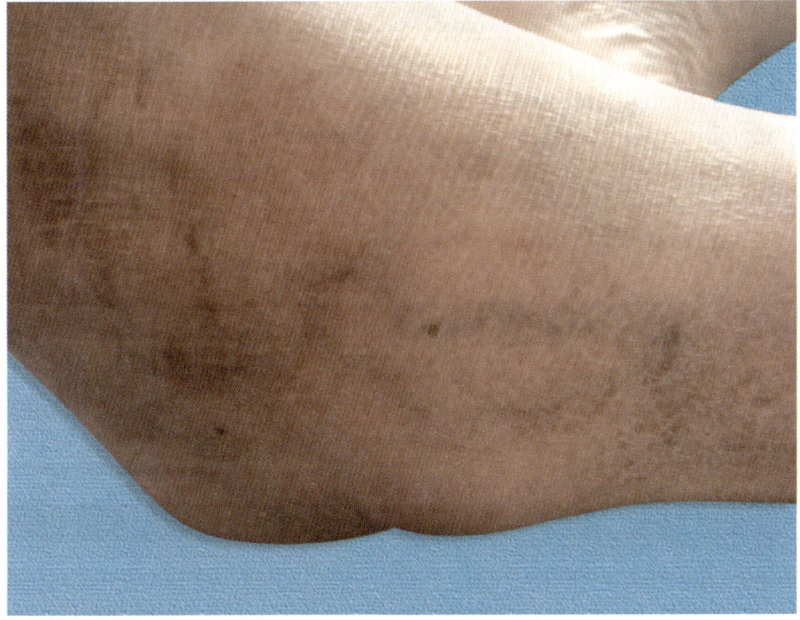

Fig. 3.2: Reticular veins.

CORONA PHLEBECTATICA PARAPLANTARIS (ANKLE FLARE)

The ankle flare is an early sign of venous insufficiency and occurs due to increased capillary pressure which causes the vessels to expand.[6]

SUPERFICIAL THROMBOPHLEBITIS

The prominence of varicose veins makes them more susceptible to local trauma which incites thrombophlebitis. Clinically it appears as tender, warm thickened area along the course of vein. Associated systemic features like fever and malaise may be present. Rarely an iliofemoral thrombus can result due to the propagation of thrombophlebitis beyond the saphenofemoral junction into the common femoral vein, which may pose a subsequent risk for pulmonary thromboembolism.

HEMORRHAGE

Bleeding from large varicosities can be either spontaneous or following minor trauma.

This is usually painless and patients might be unaware until they feel blood running down their leg. It can be managed easily by simple compression and leg elevation. Tourniquet, which is just tight enough to occlude arterial flow, can enhance venous congestion and increase the rate of hemorrhage.[7]

PIGMENTATION

Due to the prolonged venous tension resulting in venous dilation, red blood cells pass through the endothelium into the interstitium. The breakdown of hemoglobin results in hemosiderin which causes brown pigmentation on the skin. This pigmentation is typically located on the lower medial third of the leg. The pigmentation is initially minimal or patchy but may also extend to large indurated areas with time (Fig. 3.3).

PRESSURE ERYTHEMA

Pressure erythema is often the first sign of evolving venous insufficiency. Very small grouped telangiectasia develop around the incompetent perforating veins due to elevated capillary pressure.[6]

ECZEMA

Chronic inflammatory changes, fibrin and hemosiderin deposition and edema results in venous dermatitis. The eczema can be either acute or subacute. It is sharply demarcated and may be infiltrated with papules and vesicles. Scaling, itching and lichenification may develop with time. Venous ulceration can develop spontaneously with progressive loss of epithelium (Figs. 3.4 and 3.5). Contact dermatitis is more frequent in response to medications or elastic bandages.[1]

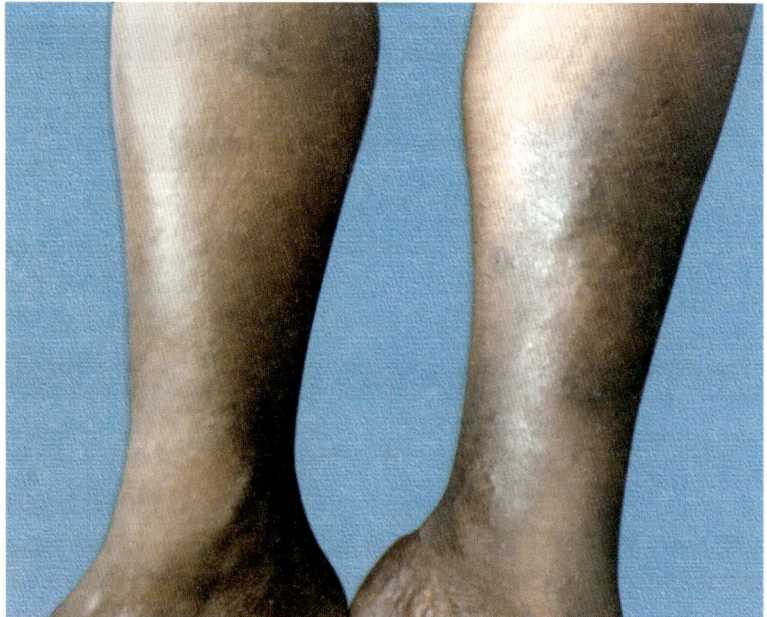

Fig. 3.3: Pigmentation of lower limbs.

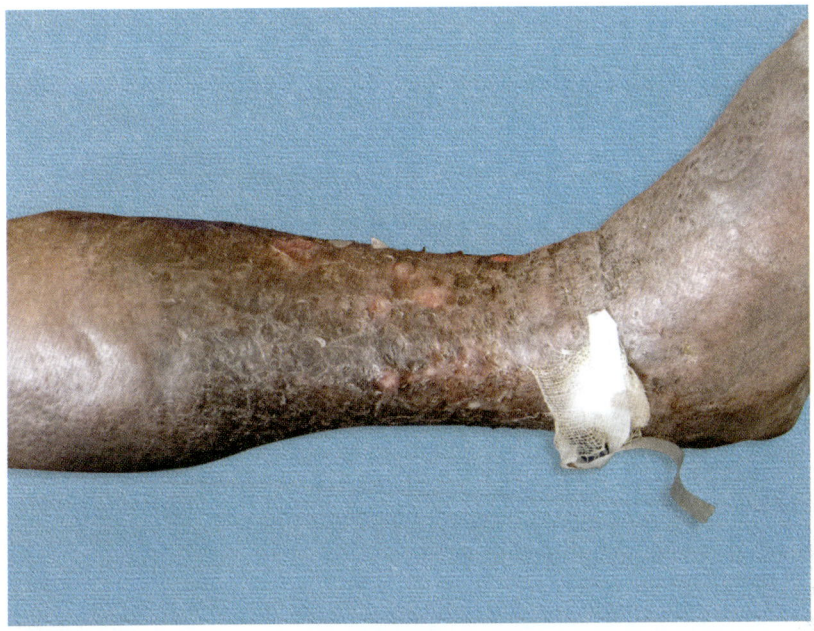

Fig. 3.4: Acute eczema.

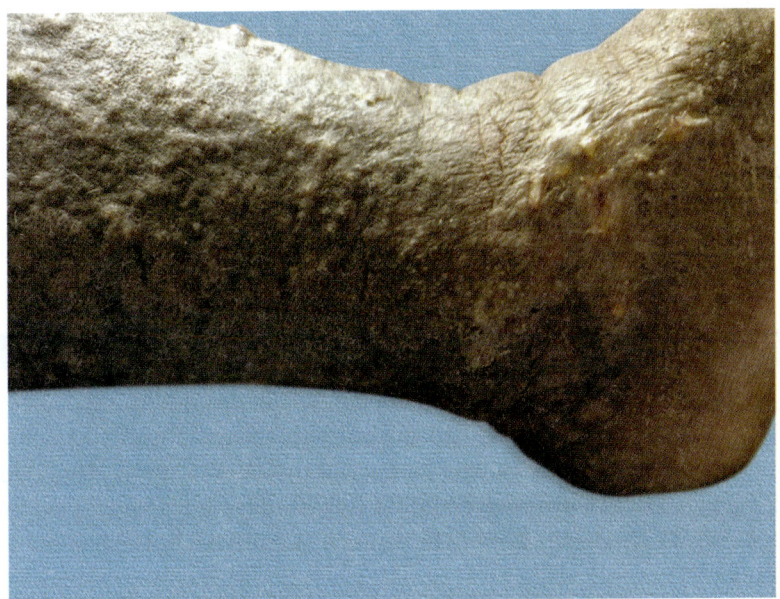

Fig. 3.5: Chronic eczema with varicose ulcer.

LIPODERMATOSCLEROSIS

Lipodermatosclerosis is progressive fibrosis of skin and subcutaneous tissue induced by chronic venous hypertension and is associated with increased

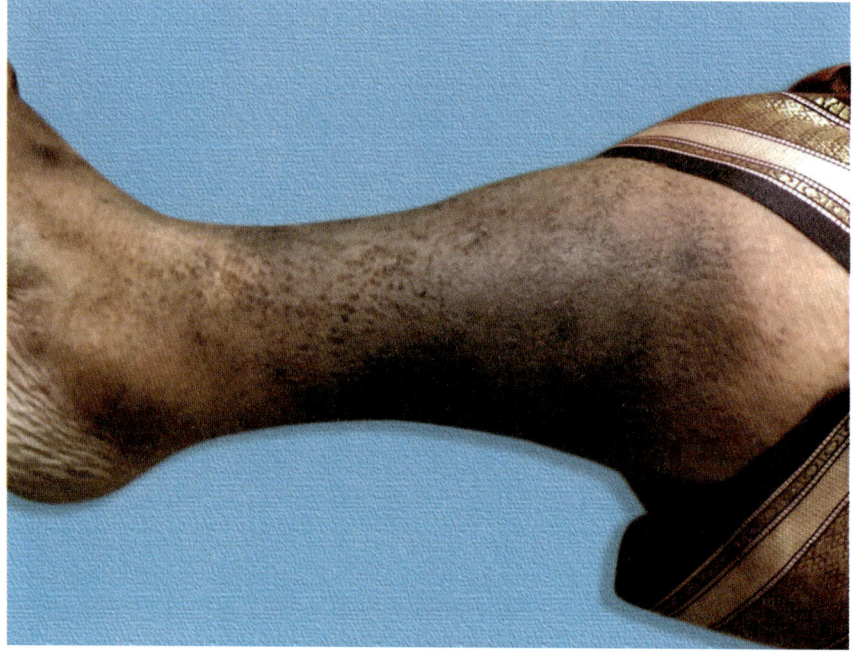

Fig. 3.6: Lipodermatosclerosis.

risk of leg ulcers. It may be either acute or chronic. The acute form eventually progresses to chronic form. Acute form appears as tender, elevated erythematous area. The differential diagnosis will be erysipelas, superficial venous thrombosis or even deep vein thrombosis. Stiff shiny skin that is fixed, hard and indurated are features of chronic lipodermatosclerosis (Fig. 3.6). Progressive contraction of the skin and subcutaneous tissues results in shrinking of the gaiter area and, accentuated by any edema in the calf above, gives the leg a stick-like or inverted bottle shape.[6]

ATROPHIE BLANCHE

Small atrophic patches of skin, few millimeter in size due to skin necrosis without ulceration healing in scars are atrophie blanche. This is an effect of reduced capillary density caused by microthrombi and matrix degradation causing hypoxia. Coalescence of multiple areas may form a large scar which may break down. Atrophie blanche as such is painless, but ulcers are very painful.[1]

ULCERATION

All the above described skin changes are pre-ulcerous. If the condition is progressive due to reduced tissue nutrition and oxygen supply, ulceration occurs. Trauma also induces ulcer.

If not treated appropriately, there could be secondary infection and necrosis which can extend deeper up to periosteum in later stages.

Mechanism of Venous Ulceration[8]

Two theories have been put forward:
1. Fibrin cuff theory
2. White cell trapping theory

Fibrin Cuff Theory

In 1982, Browse and Burnand proposed that oxygen diffusion into cutaneous tissues was restricted by a pericapillary fibrin cuff. They suggested that increased capillary pressure resulting from elevated venous pressure produces an increased loss of plasma proteins, including fibrinogen, through the capillary wall. Fibrinogen then polymerizes to produce the 'fibrin cuff' that surrounds cutaneous capillary walls. Measurements of capillary protein loss by Browse and Burnand showed that fibrinogen was quantitatively the most important plasma protein leaking into tissues in patients with venous disease. Subsequent measurements of fibrinolysis have shown that patients with venous disease have reduced venous fibrinolytic activity, which might explain why the fibrin cuff persists.

The fibrin cuff theory has tended to perpetuate the suggestions of previous authors that the nature of venous ulceration is closely related to the deprivation of oxygen in tissue.

The possibility remains that some elements in the skin may receive insufficient nutrition, which renders them susceptible to injury by mechanical or other factors.

White Cell Trapping Theory

Researchers have found that patients with venous disease were 'trapping' 30% of white blood cells and control subjects were trapping 7% on prolonged immobilization. White blood cell activation releases proteolytic enzymes, superoxide radicals and chemotactic substances. All classes of white blood cells appear to become trapped, and so a wide range of phenomena is possible. Monocytes might become activated, releasing interleukin-1 (IL-1) and TNFα. These agents may produce endothelial cell activation to permit the passage of much larger than normal molecules. Decreased fibrinolysis observed in patients with venous disease may be a result of the effects of IL-1. IL-1 acts on endothelial cells to stimulate production of the fibrinolytic inhibitor plasminogen activator inhibitor-1 (PAI-1) and decrease the production of tissue plasminogen activator (t-PA), producing a reduction in fibrinolysis.[9]

Ulceration of the lower leg is the result of persistently elevated venous pressure and its secondary effects on the microvascular system. Nearly half of all venous ulcers are associated with deep vein valvular incompetence or post-thrombotic damage while the remainder results from incompetence of the superficial or communicating veins. Venous ulcers are the end result of superficial venous insufficiency or post-thrombotic syndrome. The consequent alterations in the microvasculature and interstitium make the skin more liable to break down, or to fail to repair, following minor degrees of trauma. The fundamental fault is a sustained capillary hypertension resulting from persistently raised venous pressure. A failure to reduce venous pressure satisfactorily when the lower limb is dependent is a combination of hemodynamic failures, mainly consequent upon a failure of venous valves and poor calf muscle pump function. The skin changes resulting from venous hypertension often, but not always, culminates in ulceration.[10]

The ulcer may be preceded by patchy erythema or discoloration of intense bluish red color, in which ischemia of the skin finally leads to necrosis, often following a minor trauma. The ulcer is characteristically situated on the medial lower aspect of the leg, the gaiter region, which is drained on the medial side by three large pairs of perforating veins.

Two events may lead to a break in the continuity of surface epithelium. The first is capillary thrombosis, when the complete outline of the capillary can be seen to be filled with broken up thrombus, which does not disperse on pressure. The second is a small bleed from the peak of the capillary; this separates the epidermis from its blood supply. These changes in the capillaries supplying the epidermis are frequently induced by small knocks, scratching or epidermal pathology such as dermatitis.

The skin around an ulcer is frequently irritated by exudates, and inflamed varicose or medicament dermatitis may contribute. Ulcers often show pseudoepitheliomatous hyperplasia at their edge which may be mistaken for a squamous cell carcinoma. Healing ulcers have a shallow sloping edge with healthy granulation in their base and little slough. Non-healing ulcers resemble severe paronychia, being boggy, undermined and congested[6] (Fig. 3.7).

OTHER RARE COMPLICATIONS

Ankle Joint Stiffness

Progressive subcutaneous scarring occasionally extends into the subcutaneous tissue around the ankle joint, restricting ankle movement, reducing calf pump efficiency, and exacerbating the venous hypertension. Fibrous ankylosis may eventually fix the ankle joint with scar tissue.

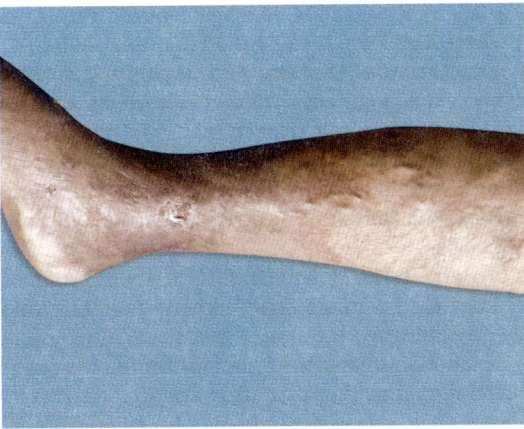

Fig. 3.7: Varicose ulcers.

Fixed Plantar Flexion

Chronic pain of acute lipodermatosclerosis or ulcer may result in abnormal weight bearing and eventually ankle stiffening and shortening of the Achilles tendon.

Periostitis

Long-standing inflammation in soft tissues may induce hyperemia in the underlying periosteum, which can then produce new subperiosteal bone. It is most often a coincidental finding on a plain radiograph.

Secondary Lymphedema

Secondary lymphedema develops when the healthy lymphatic system fails to face the increased filtration load with eventual structural obliteration of lymphatic routes.[6]

REFERENCES

1. Nicholls SC. Sequelae of untreated venous insufficiency. Semin Intervent Radiol. 2005;22(3):162-8.
2. Goldman MP, Weiss RA, Bergan JJ. Diagnosis and treatment of varicose veins: a review. J Am Acad Dermatol. 1994;31(3 Pt 1):393-413.
3. Weiss RA, Weiss MA. Treatment of varicose and telangiectatic veins. In: Freedberg JM, Eisen AZ, Wolff K, et al. (Eds). Fitzpatrick's Dermatology in General Medicine (6th edition). USA: McGraw-Hill; 2003. pp. 2549-56.
4. Das S. Disease of veins. In: A Concise Textbook of Surgery (3rd edition). SB Publications; pp. 200-9.

5. O'Leary DP, Chester JF, Jones SM. Management of varicose veins according to reason for presentation. Ann R Coll Surg Engl. 1996;78(3 Pt 1):214-6.
6. Mortimer PS, Burnand KG. Diseases of the veins and arteries: Leg ulcers, In: Burns T, Breathnach S, Cox N, et al. (Eds). Rooks Textbook of Dermatology (7th edition). Oxford, UK: Blackwell Science Ltd; 2004. pp. 1-50.
7. Harman RR. Letter: Haemorrhage from varicose veins. Lancet. 1974;1(7853):363.
8. Johnson G Jr. Management of venous disorders. In: Rutherford RB (Ed). Vascular Surgery (4th edition). Vol II. Philadelphia: WB Sounders Company; 1995. pp. 1671-862.
9. Russell RCG, Williams NS, Bulstrode CJK. Venous disorders. In: Bailey and Love's Short Practice of Surgery (24th edition). London: Arnold Publications; 2004. pp. 954-73.
10. Valencia IC, Falabella A, Kirsner RS, et al. Chronic venous insufficiency and venous leg ulceration. J Am Acad Dermatol. 2001;44(3):401-21; quiz 422-4.

CHAPTER 4

Evaluation of Varicose Veins

Shilpa K, Lakshmi DV, Divya Gorur K

INTRODUCTION

Chronic venous insufficiency is a complex and chronic condition, with varied clinical manifestations, etiologies and underlying pathophysiology. A thorough stepwise workup is essential to assess the nature of a patient's underlying venous disease. This should begin in the clinical setting itself with a careful medical history, physical examination and bedside diagnostic tests. These need to be supplemented by confirmatory diagnostic testing, including duplex ultrasonography, venography, plethysmography and ambulatory venous pressure measurement. Based upon the results of these examinations, venous disease can be classified according to standardized classification schemes, which in turn helps in selection of an appropriate treatment strategy.

HISTORY

Initial evaluation should begin in the office setting with a thorough history. The history should include:
- Symptoms suggestive of venous insufficiency (Box 4.1)
- Worsening of symptoms during the course of the day and with prolonged standing
- Specific features of the pain that should be noted include the degree to which the pain interferes with the patient's occupation or lifestyle
- The duration of time the patient can stand before the onset of pain or swelling
- The age of onset of varicose veins should be recorded (early onset in congenital abnormality such as Klippel–Trenaunay syndrome)
- History of deep vein thrombosis or pulmonary embolism
- History of past treatments for varicose veins, including operative and percutaneous procedures

A proper history should be followed by thorough physical examination which includes general physical examination along with careful examination of lower extremities.

Box 4.1: Symptoms suggestive of venous insufficiency.
- Pain
- Tightness
- Skin irritation
- Pruritus
- Heaviness
- Tingling
- Muscle cramps
- Cosmetically unacceptable linear swellings
- Edema
- Skin pigmentation
- Ulceration

Prerequisites

- Examination should be done in a well-lit and warm room
- Patient should be examined in standing position
- It is suitable to undress the patient allowing complete exposure of lower limbs from groin to toes

Examination

Inspection

The location and distribution of all major subcutaneous varicosities should be noted. The findings should be recorded using charts or line diagrams. Large varicosities especially over the anatomical areas of perforators should be noted. Presence or absence of edema, vascular malformation should be noted. Spider veins if any should be recorded. Cutaneous changes like pigmentation, scars, atrophie blanche, lipodermatosclerosis, ulceration (Figs. 4.1A to C) should be documented.

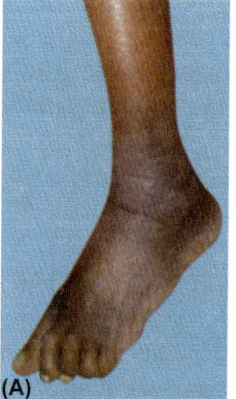
(A)
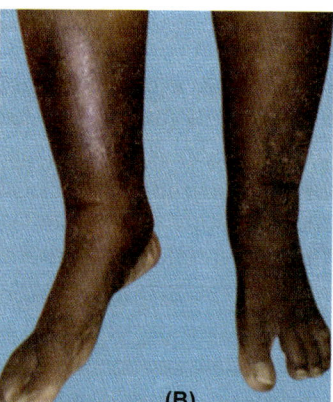
(B)
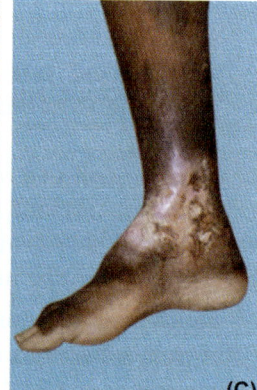
(C)

Figs. 4.1A to C: Cutaneous changes due to varicose veins, (A) pigmentation, (B) lipodermatosclerosis and (C) healing ulcer with scarring and depigmentation.

Palpation

All the inspectory findings should be confirmed by palpation. Palpation of the limbs may detect additional varicosities that are not readily appreciated by inspection especially the terminal segments of the greater saphenous vein (GSV) (inner thigh) and lesser saphenous vein (LSV) (calf) where they join the femoral and popliteal veins, respectively. Palpation also throws light on presence of areas of induration, firm subcutaneous cords (due to previous episodes of thrombophlebitis) and presence of temperature difference between the legs.

BEDSIDE TESTS

Cough Impulse Test[1,2]

This test is performed while the patient is in standing position. Proximal part of the thigh at fossa ovalis (Fig. 4.2) is palpated and the patient is asked to cough. A palpable thrill at the saphenofemoral junction (SFJ), as a result of turbulent retrograde flow, indicates reflux at the SFJ. The drawback of the test is, it is difficult to perform in obese individuals.

Tap Test or Percussion Test[3,4]

This test is also performed while palpating the SFJ in standing position. The GSV is tapped at the level of the knee. A palpable transmitted impulse at the SFJ suggests that the GSV is distended with blood. Conversely, the SFJ is then tapped while the GSV is palpated at the knee. A palpable transmitted pulse at

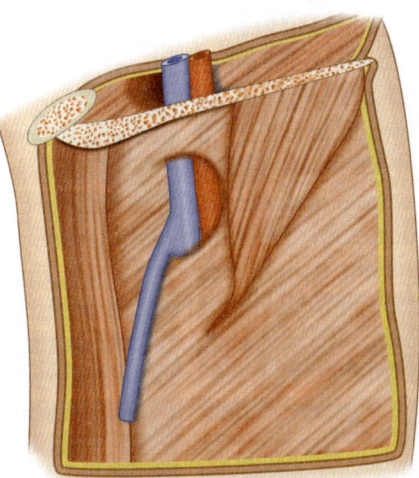

Fig. 4.2: Fossa ovalis an oval opening in the upper mid-part of the fascia lata of the thigh which lies 3–4 cm below and lateral to the pubic tubercle and is about 3 cm long and 1.5 cm wide and transmits great saphenous vein.

the knee with this maneuver indicates incompetence of GSV valves between the SFJ and the knee.[4]

Brodie-Trendelenburg Test[5]

Brodie-Trendelenburg test is done to differentiate between perforator and GSV incompetence. The Brodie-Trendelenburg test is highly sensitive for the identification of superficial and perforator reflux (91%), although poorly specific (15%).[4] The test is performed with patient in supine position. First the superficial lower extremity veins are drained by raising the lower limbs to 45° and gently stroking the limb along the course of the major veins from foot towards thigh. A tourniquet is applied as close to the groin as possible and tight enough to prevent reflux in superficial veins. Then the patient is made to stand and leg is examined for refilling of veins (Fig. 4.3). If the distal veins remain collapsed for 15 to 30 seconds after standing, the tourniquet is released.[6] Interpretation of the test is given in the Table 4.1.

Modified Trendelenburg Test

In this test, firstly, the leg is elevated and the veins are emptied. The tourniquet is applied to control the saphenous vein near fossa ovalis. The patient then stands up and the tourniquet is removed at once. The sudden filling of

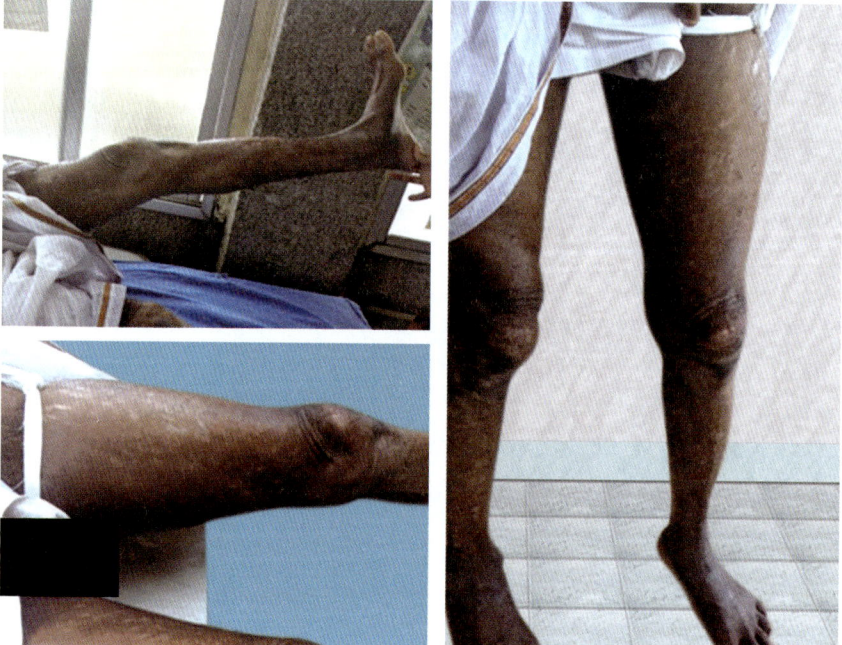

Fig. 4.3: Demonstration of Brodie-Trendelenburg test.

Evaluation of Varicose Veins

Table 4.1: Interpretation of Brodie-Trendelenburg test.

Observation	Inference
If the caudal veins fill rapidly when the patient stands with the tourniquet in place	Perforator incompetence is suggested
The location of the incompetent perforator can then be determined by varying the position of the tourniquet	
Rapid filling of the varices with a tourniquet in the suprapatellar position	Incompetent mid-thigh perforator
Rapid filling with the tourniquet below the knee	Incompetent lower leg perforators
If the distal veins fill rapidly upon release of the tourniquet	SFJ incompetence

varicose veins from above down indicates a reflex through a saphenous femoral valve and valvular incompetence.[7]

Perthes Test[8]

Perthes test is highly sensitive but poorly specific similar to Trendelenburg test. It is performed with the patient in standing position with a tourniquet positioned below the knee (Fig. 4.4). The patient is asked to raise heel ten times to activate the calf muscle pump.[8] Interpretation of Perthes test is given in Table 4.2.

Modified Perthes Test

The leg is elevated and the veins are emptied. A tourniquet is applied to the upper thigh to constrict the saphenous vein return flow. The patient then walks around the room for five minutes. Absence of pain in the calf or definite swelling of the foot and ankle indicates patent deep veins.[3]

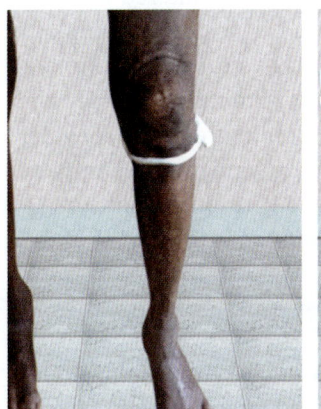 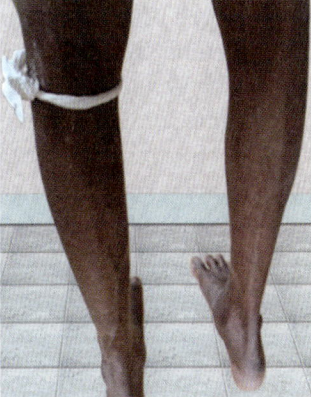

Fig. 4.4: Demonstration of Perthes test.

Table 4.2: Interpretation of Perthes test.	
Observation	Inference
Emptying of the varicose veins	The site of reflux is cranial to the tourniquet, namely the SFJ, saphenopopliteal junction (SPJ), or thigh perforators
Persistence of distended varicose veins	The site of reflux caudal to the tourniquet, that is, calf perforators
Pain associated with heel raising	It suggests the possibility of deep venous obstruction

Validation of Bedside Tests in Varicose Veins

A validation study conducted by Kim J et al. to determine the accuracy of clinical tests compared to color duplex imaging in patients with primary varicose veins using a prospective, blinded comparison study showed that the cough test had low sensitivity (0.59) and specificity (0.67). The tap test had low sensitivity (0.18) and high specificity (0.92). The Trendelenburg test had high sensitivity (0.91) but low specificity (0.15), and Perthes test had a high sensitivity (0.97) but low specificity (0.20). Hand-held Doppler assessment of reflux at the SFJ, in the long saphenous vein and at the SPJ had high sensitivity (0.97, 0.82 and 0.80 respectively) and specificity (0.73, 0.92 and 0.90 respectively) of detecting reflux. They also concluded that clinical tests used in the examination of patients with primary varicose veins are inaccurate.[1]

IMAGING STUDIES

Clinical evaluation based on the distribution of the venous abnormality can suggest a pattern of incompetence. However, treatment decisions based solely upon clinical evaluations are often encountered with errors, as several different patterns of incompetence can result in a similar appearance of abnormalities clinically. Therefore, it is strongly recommended that all patients undergoing evaluation for lower extremity varicose veins should be subjected to imaging studies before planning treatment. Several modalities have been used for this purpose including venography, Doppler ultrasound, computed tomography (CT), and magnetic resonance imaging (MRI); however, all of these methods have limitations.

Venography

Venography is a procedure in which a special dye is injected into the veins followed by X-ray of the veins, called a venogram, is taken (Fig. 4.5).[9] The dye has to be injected constantly via a catheter, making it an invasive procedure.

Evaluation of Varicose Veins 35

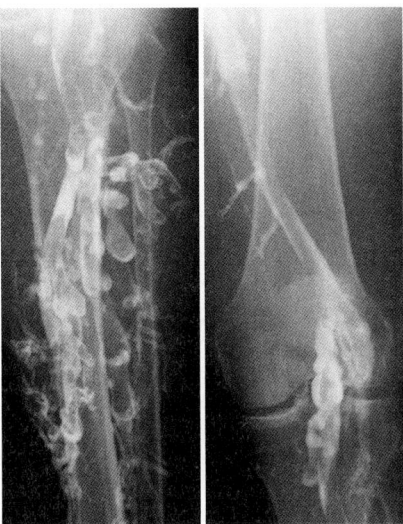

Fig. 4.5: Venogram, taken after injecting special dye into the veins followed by X-ray of the veins.

Normally the catheter is inserted in the groin and moved to the appropriate site by navigating through the vascular system.

Contrast venography[10] is the gold standard for judging diagnostic imaging methods for deep venous thrombosis although; because of its cost, invasiveness, and other limitations this test is rarely performed.

Venography gives an image of the entire length of the lower extremity veins; yet, the image may often be inadequate despite the use of a large volume of contrast medium. Hence, this diagnostic technique is not advocated nowadays.

Doppler Ultrasound[11,12]

Duplex ultrasonography (DUS) is an essential part of the evaluation of patients with most forms of superficial venous insufficiency (Figs. 4.6A and B). Although other techniques exist, DUS is an inexpensive, portable and reproducible means of simultaneously assessing both the venous anatomy and physiology.

Indication

Patients undergoing evaluation for lower extremity varicose veins edema, or venous cutaneous changes (CEAP clinical stage 2-6) should also undergo an ultrasound evaluation of the superficial venous system to determine the pattern(s) of incompetence prior to making treatment recommendations. Patients with spider veins (CEAP clinical stage 1), particularly those in typical distributions such as on the lateral thigh area, generally do not require US evaluation. However, when the spider veins are found in the distribution of

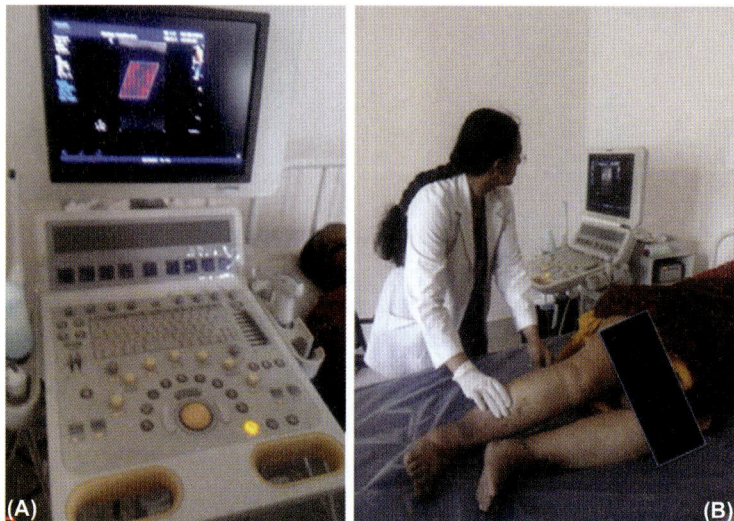

Figs. 4.6A and B: (A) Doppler ultrasound machine and (B) examination of veins.

a large truncal veins such as the GSV, it is recommended that DUS be performed. If truncal vein reflux is identified and contributory in these cases, treatment of reflux may be warranted prior to treatment of the spider veins.[13]

Procedure

When evaluating patients for reflux, the examination should be performed in the standing position. The patient is usually positioned on a stand to elevate the legs, which facilitates the performance of the examination. The patient is asked to turn the leg under examination, outward to allow scanning of the inner thigh and calf. Generally, the examination begins at the SFJ (Fig. 4.7). Further the great saphenous veins and short saphenous veins are followed downwards tracing their course and also the course of any tributaries that might lead to the abnormal veins. Competence of perforators are also evaluated (Fig. 4.8). It is important to be aware of the standard tributary anatomy of the GSV and to recognize the frequent variations that are found.

Doppler ultrasound is noninvasive and provides morphological and hemodynamic information, but it takes time for scanning the entire leg, and the accuracy and quality of assessment depends on the skill of the assessor/radiologist.

Still, Doppler ultrasound is the most recommended and widely performed diagnostic procedure in evaluation of varicose veins.

Ambulatory Venous Pressure

Ambulatory venous pressure (AVP) is the test of the efficiency of the calf musculovenous pump.[14]

Evaluation of Varicose Veins **37**

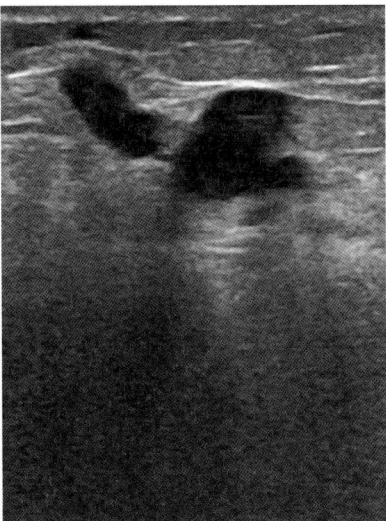

Fig. 4.7: Doppler ultrasonography showing SFJ (Real time B mode image).

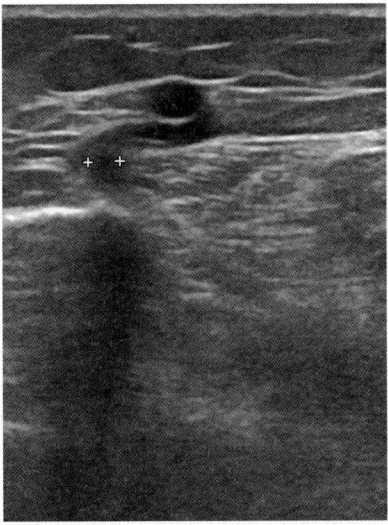

Fig. 4.8: Doppler ultrasonography showing perforator incompetence (Real time B mode image).

Procedure

A small needle is placed into one of the veins on the back of the foot and the needle is connected to a blood pressure measurement machine. The subject is then asked to stand up and the standing venous pressure is measured. In a normal subject, the standing venous pressure is around 90 mm Hg. The subject is then asked to perform ten heel raise exercises to work the musculovenous

Table 4.3: Interpretation of Ambulatory venous pressure (AVP) test.	
Observation	Inference
No fall in the pressure	Indicates that the calf pump is not working effectively
Pressure rises rather than to fall during exercise	Indicates that the deep veins occlusion
AVP returns to the standing pressure too quickly	Indicates reflux in either the deep or superficial veins due to absent or damaged valves

pump during which AVP is recorded. During exercise, this should fall to around 30 mm Hg. Later, the subject is asked to rest again in the standing position and the rate at which the ambulatory pressure returns to the standing pressure is measured, called the refilling time. Normally, after exercise, the fallen AVP should rise slowly over half a minute or so back to the standing pressure.

Results are analyzed as in Table 4.3.

Ambulatory venous pressure measurement is a specialist, invasive test which is only performed in patients with clinical evidence of chronic venous insufficiency (CEAP 3-6). Photoplethysmography is used as an alternative in patients with varicose veins only (CEAP 2).

Plethysmography

Plethysmography is a noninvasive test that measures and records the variations in volume and pressure as blood flows through the tissues.[15] In diagnosing varicose veins and CVD, either strain gauge plethysmography or air plethysmography is used to evaluate the function of the calf muscle, global venous reflux, and obstructions to venous outflow. Gloviczki et al.[16] stated that although venous plethysmography is not used as often for patients suffering from simple varicose veins, the test can be used for patients who have more advanced stages of varicose veins and CVD, and is considered complementary to venous duplex scanning when venous reflux or outflow obstruction is suspected but is not visualized with the duplex scan.

Computed Tomography[17]

Though Doppler ultrasonography (US) has been used for evaluation of varicose veins, computed tomographic venography is useful when varicose veins arise from an unexpected anatomic source (Fig. 4.9). CT can provide an overview of the varicose veins in these cases.

Doppler US with complementary CT venography is useful for determining the precise cause of varicose veins. The use of CT venography aids in the overall understanding of varicosities and suspicious causes. The radiologist

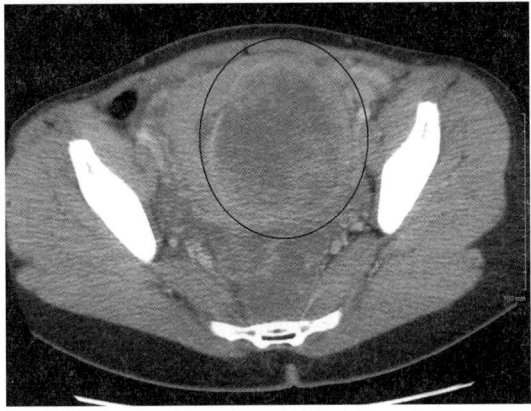

Fig. 4.9: CT scan showing pelvic vascular lesion causing varicose veins due to pressure effects.

can evaluate varicosities and determine their precise cause in most cases, particularly in unusual causes, with the combined strategy of Doppler US and CT venography is used.[14]

Magnetic Resonance Imaging

Magnetic resonance imaging is rarely indicated for patients who present with simple varicose veins because duplex scanning is usually enough to locate any obstructions or venous abnormalities. However, MRI may be helpful in identifying obstructions in the pelvic venous system or the iliac vein when proximal obstructions are suspected.[18] These tests can identify left renal vein compression, gonadal vein incompetence and pelvic venous congestion syndrome, and MRI with gadolinium contrast is helpful in evaluating CVD in patients with vascular malformations, such as congenital varicose veins.

CONCLUSION

Dermatologist often encounter with cases of varicose veins due to their varied cutaneous manifestations. Though good history, clinical examination, bedside tests can suggest a pattern of incompetence; they need to be confirmed by imaging studies especially when a therapeutic intervention is planned. Doppler being inexpensive, portable and reproducible mode of diagnostic technique is the most recommended and preferred method in evaluation of varicose veins. CT and MRI rarely indicated for patients who present with simple varicose veins, only useful when varicose veins arise from an unexpected anatomic source or identifying obstructions in the pelvic venous system or the iliac vein or when proximal obstructions are suspected.

REFERENCES

1. Jones RH, Carek PJ. Management of varicose veins. Am Fam Physician. 2008; 78(11):1289-94.
2. Dodd H. Diagnosis of varicose veins. Postgrad Med J. 1947;23(263):427-40.
3. Pedrycz A, Budzyńska B. Diagnosis of varicose veins of the lower limbs-funtional tests. Arch Physiother Glob Res. 2016;20(3):29-32.
4. Kim J, Richards S, Kent PJ. Clinical examination of varicose veins: a validation study. Ann R Coll Surg Engl. 2000;82(3):171-5.
5. Browse NL, Burnand KG, Irvine AT, et al. Diseases of the Veins (2nd edition). London: Arnold Publishers; 1999. pp. 169-89.
6. Krishnan S, Nicholls SC. Chronic venous insufficiency: clinical assessment and patient selection. Semin Intervent Radiol. 2005;22(3):169-77.
7. Pratt GH. Test for incompetent communicating branches in the surgical treatment of varicose veins. JAMA. 1941;117(2):100-1.
8. Devi AS, Aathi MK. Prevention of varicose veins. Int J Adv Nur Management. 2014;2(1):40-5. J Nur Sci Prac. 2014;4(1):23-9.
9. Muir IF, Muklow EH, Rains AJ. Venography and the approach to varicose veins. Br J Sur. 1954;42(173):276-82.
10. Naidich JB, Feinberg AW, Karp-Harman H, et al. Contrast venography: reassessment of its role. Radiology. 1988;168(1):97-100.
11. Jung SC, Lee W, Chung JW, et al. Unusual causes of varicose veins in the lower extremities: CT venographic and Doppler US findings. Radiographics. 2009;29(2): 525-36.
12. Meissner MH, Moneta G, Burnand K, et al. The hemodynamics and diagnosis of venous disease. J Vasc Sur. 2007;46(6):S4-S24.
13. Khilnani NM, Min RJ. Imaging of venous insufficiency. Semin Intervent Radiol. 2005;22(3):178-84.
14. Dix FP, McCollum CN. Role of ambulatory venous pressure measurement in the assessment of venous disease. Phlebology. 2003;18:23-9.
15. Roberts D. Nursing assessment: musculoskeletal system. In: Lewis SL, Dirksen SR, Heitkemper MM, et al. (Eds). Medical-Surgical Nursing: Assessment and Management of Clinical Problems (8th edition). St Louis, MO: Mosby; 2011. pp. 1568-82.
16. Gloviczki P, Comerota AJ, Dalsing MC, et al. The care of patients with varicose veins and associated chronic venous diseases: clinical practice guidelines of the Society for Vascular Surgery and the American Venous Forum. J Vasc Surg. 2011;53(5):2S-48S.
17. Min SK, Kim SY, Park YJ, et al. Role of three-dimensional computed tomography venography as a powerful navigator for varicose vein surgery. J Vasc Surg. 2010;51(4):893-9.

CHAPTER 5

Compression Therapy following Sclerotherapy

Late GR Ratnavel

INTRODUCTION

Sclerotherapy is a form of chemical ablation where, a sclerosing solution is injected into an abnormal vessel. Sclerotherapy causes endothelial destruction, resulting in inflammation and then collapse, and shut down of the vascular structure. The cornerstone of treatment for varicose veins and other vascular and lymphatic malformations is correctly applied compression therapy following the sclerotherapy.

COMPRESSION THERAPY

Mechanism of Action of Compressive Therapy in Varicose Veins[1,2]

People with varicose veins tend to have a higher venous pressure during rising and walking as compared with the normal individuals due to the pooling of blood (Fig. 5.1). Compression therapy in general, has the following mechanisms of action,
- Provides a static effect or resting pressure and a dynamic effect due to the changing circumference of the leg during walking.
- Increases the limb pressure, which, according to Pascal's Law, will be distributed evenly.
- Prevents pooling of fluid in the limb—the amount of fluid pushed out being proportionate to the amount of pressure applied.
- Prevents leakage of blood into surface venous system during calf muscle contraction, so it will not leak out to the superficial system.

by which it reduces the venous pressure by pushing out the stasis fluid.

Properties of an Ideal Compression System

- Conformable, i.e., produces a good anatomical fit
- Allows full functionality and movement
- Easy to apply and adapt to a range of limb sizes and shapes
- Non-allergic and durable

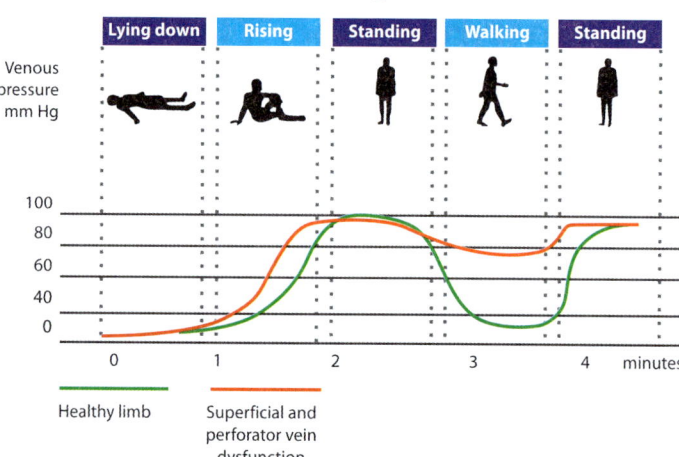

Fig. 5.1: Changes in pressure (measured at the ankle) in the venous system in legs with healthy and defective venous valves during lying, rising, standing and exercise.

Types of Compression Therapy

- *Compression bandages:* Long strips of fabric that are wrapped around the leg to form a continuous covering.
- *Multi-layer bandaging systems* (e.g., four-layers and two layers): Bandages which are applied in layers usually with additional materials such as padding.
- *Compression hosiery (stockings):* Knitted garments that have anatomical shaping and are applied like a piece of clothing.
- *Elastic (long stretch) compression:* Contain elastic (elastomeric) fibers which can be stretched to increase the overall length of the material by over 100%. They return to their original length when the tension is released.
- *Inelastic (short stretch) compression:* Contain few or no elastic fibers and increase in length by less than 100% when stretched.[3]

Pressure Applied

According to the pressure produced on a model limb at the ankle during laboratory testing, compression bandage systems can be categorized as given below[4] (Fig. 5.2).

Ideal pressure for compression hosiery for preventing venous leg ulcer is 18–24 mm Hg and up to 35 mm Hg at the ankle.[5]

Static Stiffness Index

Measured by recording the pressure at the interface between the compression therapy system and the skin (the interface pressure), when the patient is

Category	Pressure
Mild	<20mmHg
Moderate	≥20–40 mm Hg
Strong	≥40–60 mm Hg
Very strong	≥60 mm Hg

Fig. 5.2: Categories according to pressure.

lying down and when they are standing.[6] Static stiffness index (SSI) is the difference between the two measurements. Compression therapy systems with a high SSI (inelastic or multi-layer bandage system) will produce higher pressures during standing, and lower pressures when lying down than systems with a lower SSI (an elastic system).

Rationale for using Compression Bandage after Sclerotherapy

Compression after sclerotherapy[7] leads to:
- More effective fibrosis
- Decreased thrombus formation
- Decreased extent of thrombus into the deep venous system
- Reduced level of discomfort

TYPES OF COMPRESSION AFTER SCLEROTHERAPY

- Local permanent compression with cotton pads or rolls after injection
- Digital short-term compression of the injected site

Graduated Compression Stockings

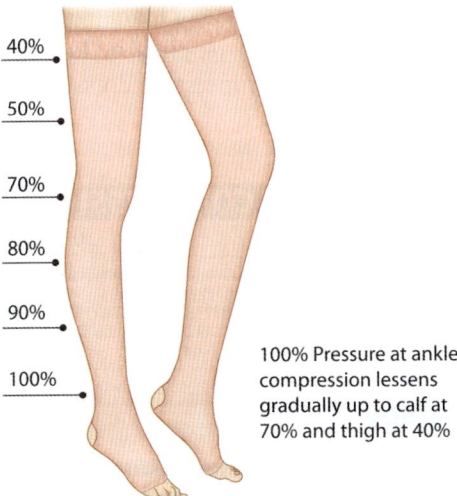

100% Pressure at ankle, compression lessens gradually up to calf at 70% and thigh at 40%

Fig. 5.3: Percentage of pressure at various levels with compression stockings.

- Compression or intermittent compression with duplex probe
- Permanent elastic compression with bandages or stockings

WHAT DO GUIDELINES AND STUDIES SAY

American venous forum recommends a compression therapy for a minimum period of 1 week after injection sclerotherapy with compression bandages or stockings.[7]

Neumann in 1999 studied 100 patients and 120 legs who underwent sclerotherapy of large veins, and were treated with cotton rolls and elastic stockings. There were good clinical results in all patients, and only three patients needed incision and thrombus expression.[8]

Schadek[9] used intermittent compression by duplex probe after injecting a saphenous vein until there was reduction in the diameter of the vein. He demonstrated better results without the use of elastic permanent compression. Intermittent compression with duplex probe increased the venospasm after sclerotherapy.

Batch et al.[10] in 1980 showed that there was no significant difference in results or complication among the 148 patients who were injected using Fegan technique and followed up for 2 years.

Weiss et al.[11] showed no significant differences in matting, bruising, edema and ulceration in patients who did not use compression (n = 10) and those who used 3 days (n = 10), 1 week (n = 10) and 3 weeks (n = 10) of compression after sclerotherapy.

About 30 mm Hg support stockings for 3 weeks postsclerotherapy has been found to be not only effective for closing veins, immediately post injection, but also for better long-term outcome.

In a case report by G Sharma, a case of hemangioma of the glans penis, a postsclerotherapy compression was applied by local compression of the lesion for 5 minutes, followed by compression dressing application over the lesion, which was kept for 48 hours.[12]

TIME OF APPLICATION OF COMPRESSION BANDAGE

Liquid Sclerotherapy

In liquid sclerotherapy, immediate external compression leads to better contact of sclerosing agent and the venous wall.

Foam Sclerotherapy

In foam sclerotherapy, spontaneous venospasm occurs after injection. In the horizontal position of the leg, foam stays stable in the injected area of the vein. Application of external compression immediately would dislodge the foam column. Polidocanol binds to protein fraction and gets inactivated and the venous spasm resolves spontaneously after sometime. Hence, it is advised to wait for few minutes after injecting foam (before the patient is allowed to stand up).[13]

In the author's personal experience, foam sclerotherapy using sodium tetradecyl sulfate where foaming is done by Tessari method is practiced. Postsclerotherapy, compression bandaging with a moderate pressure of 20–40 mm Hg is applied starting a few minutes postsclerotherapy, in the form of stockings in affordable patients and elastocrepe bandaging in unaffordable patients, which is to be worn for 2 weeks. The patients are advised to be ambulant, to keep their legs elevated, to avoid strenuous exercise and standing still for long periods.[14]

CONCLUSION

Compression therapy appears scientific in preventing complications, and hence, the authors advocate regular postsclerotherapy compression bandages in both regular and foam sclerotherapy methods.

REFERENCES

1. O'Meara S, Cullum N, Nelson EA, et al. Compression for venous leg ulcers. Cochrane Database Syst Rev. 2012;11:CD000265.
2. Nelson EA, Bell-Syer SE. Compression for preventing recurrence of venous ulcers. Cochrane Database Syst Rev. 2014;(9):CD002303.
3. Partsch H, Clark M, Mosti G, et al. Classification of compression bandages: practical aspects. Dermatol Surg. 2008;34(5):600-9.
4. World Union of Wound Healing Societies (WUWHS). Principles of best practice: compression in venous leg ulcers. A consensus document. London: MEP Ltd; 2008.
5. Moffatt C. Compression Therapy in Practice. Wounds UK: Aberdeen; 2007.
6. Partsch H. The static stiffness index: a simple method to assess the elastic property of compression material in vivo. Dermatol Surg. 2005;31(6):625-30.
7. Villavicencio L. Handbook of Venous Disorders. UK: Chapman and Hall Medical; 1996. pp. 337-54.
8. Tazelaar DJ, Neumann HA, De Roos KP. Long cotton wool rolls as compression enhancers in macrosclerotherapy for varicose veins. Dermatol Surg. 1999;25(1):38-40.
9. Schadeck M. Echo-sclerotherapy. Phlebologie. 1999;52:103-6.
10. Batch AJ, Wickremesinghe SS, Gannon ME, et al. Randomised trial of bandaging after sclerotherapy for varicose veins. Br Med J. 1980;281(6237):423.
11. Weiss RA, Sadick NS, Goldman MP, et al. Postsclerotherapy compression: controlled comparative study of duration of compression and its effects on clinical outcome. Dermatol Surg. 1999;25(2):105-8.
12. Sharma G. Hemangioma of glans penis. Internet J Urol. 2004;3:1.
13. Breu FX, Guggenbichler S. European Consensus Meeting on Foam Sclerotherapy, April, 4-6, 2003, Tegernsee, Germany. Dermatol Surg. 2004;30(5):709-17.
14. Ratnavel GR. Foam sclerotherapy in various vascular and lymphatic malformations. Indian J Dermatol Venereol Leprol. 2011;77(3):336-8.

Chapter 6

Sclerosing Solutions

Akhilesh A

INTRODUCTION

The purpose of sclerotherapy is to produce endothelial damage that results in permanent endofibrosis and clinical obliteration of the vessel. This can be achieved by a substance called sclerosant. The sclerotherapist should have a sound knowledge of the mechanism of action, and the adverse effects of all available sclerosants in order to select the solution that will optimize results in each patient.[1]

GENERAL MECHANISM OF ACTION OF SCLEROSANTS

For an agent to have potential as a sclerosant, it must have a physical, chemical and/or biologic effect on the target tissue and induce a controlled inflammatory response. The inflammatory response is a result of cell damage with fibroblast proliferation that leads to sclerosis.[2]

The mechanism of action for sclerosing solutions is that of producing endothelial damage (endosclerosis) that causes endofibrosis. The extent of damage to the blood vessel wall determines the effectiveness of the solution.

Endothelial damage can be provoked by a number of mechanisms, such as a change in the surface tension of the plasma membrane or modification of the physical–chemical milieu of the endothelial cell through a change of intravascular pH or osmolality. The endothelium can be destroyed directly by caustic chemicals or by other physical factors such as heat and cold. For sclerotherapy to be effective without recanalization of the thrombotic vessel, the endothelial damage and resulting vascular necrosis must be extensive enough to destroy the entire blood vessel wall. Destruction of the entire vessel wall and not just the endothelium is necessary. The reason may relate to the multifunctional nature of vascular smooth muscle cells. These cells, which are found in significant concentration within superficial veins, have a large number of functions, including the synthesis of collagen, elastin and proteoglycans. It is hypothesized that if they remain viable, they can regenerate a foundation that promotes migration of undamaged adjacent endothelial cells that allow recanalization of the treated vessel.[3]

> **Table 6.1:** Sclerosing agents.[4]
>
> - *Detergents:* Disrupt vein cellular membrane (protein theft denaturation)
>   - Sodium tetradecyl sulfate
>   - Polidocanol
>   - Sodium morrhuate
>   - Ethanolamine oleate
> - *Osmotic agents:* Damage the cell by shifting the water balance
>   - Hypertonic sodium chloride solution
>   - Sodium chloride solution with dextrose
> - *Chemical irritants:* Damage the cell wall by direct caustic destruction of endothelium
>   - Chromated glycerin
>   - Polyiodinated iodine
>   - Ethanol
>   - OK 432
>   - Bleomycin

In addition, for effective destruction of a varicosity or telangiectasia, the entire vessel must be sclerosed to prevent recanalization. Recanalization occurs easily in vessels where only a section of endothelium is damaged. This is due to rapid endothelial regeneration.[3]

Total endothelial destruction results in the exposure of subendothelial collagen fibers, causing platelet aggregation, adherence and release of platelet-related factors. This series of events initiates the intrinsic pathway of blood coagulation by activating factor XII. Ideally, sclerosing solutions otherwise should not cause activation or release of thromboplastic activity because this would initiate the extrinsic pathway of blood coagulation. Excessive thrombosis is detrimental to the production of endofibrosis because it may lead to recanalization of the vessel as well as excessive intravascular and perivascular inflammation and its resulting sequelae. Therefore, endothelial damage must be complete and should result in minimal thrombus formation with subsequent organization and fibrosis.[3]

Categories of sclerosing agents are given in Table 6.1.

DETERGENTS

Mechanism of Action

Detergent solutions are the most versatile and effective sclerosants available with a capacity to treat all vein sizes. Their intravascular action causes cell surface membrane disruption and extraction of cell surface proteins within seconds and its effect continues on for minutes to hours.[5]

Because the hydrophilic and hydrophobic poles of the detergent molecule orient themselves so that the polar hydrophilic part is within the water and the hydrophobic part is away from the water, they appear as aggregates in solution (micelles) or fixed onto the endothelial surface. Because the practitioner cannot ensure that the solution is entirely in contact with the endothelial surface (if the injected vein contains blood), the decrease in surface tension on the endothelial cells may not be in direct proportion to the concentration of the solution. Strong detergent sclerosants therefore have a low safety margin.[3]

Sodium Tetradecyl Sulfate

Sodium tetradecyl sulfate is a synthetic surface-acting substance. It is a long chain fatty acid set of an alkali metal with the property of a soap. It is a clear, nonviscous liquid with low surface tension. It is composed of sodium-1 isobutyl-4 ethyl octyl sulfate plus benzoyl alcohol 2% (as an anesthetic agent) and phosphate buffered to a pH of 7.6.[6] When injected into the vessel it causes sludging of RBCs, thrombosis, intimal necrosis and luminal collapse.[7]

Sodium tetradecyl sulfate was first described in 1946,[8] and Fegan[9] popularized it for the treatment of varicose veins. Commercially available sodium tetradecyl sulfate preparations include 1% or 3% solutions, with common total dosing of 0.5 mL to 2 (although use of up to 6 mL during a single session has been reported).

It is a detergent sclerosant approved by the Food and Drug Administration (FDA) (March 2004) and is approved specifically for superficial varicosities. There have also been reports of sodium tetradecyl sulfate administration in the treatment of varicoceles, vascular malformations of the extremities, upper gastrointestinal bleeding, variceal bleeding, hemorrhagic tumors, gallbladder ablation, lymphoceles and percutaneous ablation of oral lesions of Kaposi sarcoma and ganglion cysts.[5,10,11]

Advantages

- Effective at low concentrations
- Less cytotoxic than ethanol
- Less painful/painless with intravascular injection
- Lower rates of systemic side effects
- FDA approved

Disadvantages

- Postsclerotherapy hyperpigmentation can occur (pigmentation in proportion to its concentration therefore its dilution is critical)
- Epidermal necrosis frequently occurs with extravasation of concentrations higher than 1%
- Allergic reactions occur rarely (shock and cardiorespiratory arrest)

Polidocanol

Polidocanol is composed of a mixture of hydroxypolyethoxydodecane dissolved in distilled water, to which 96% ethyl alcohol is added to a concentration of 5% to ensure emulsification of polidocanol micelles (which provides a clear solution) and to decrease foaming during the production process. Thus, 1 mL of polidocanol contains 40.5 mg of ethanol, and patients taking disulfiram should be warned about a possible alcohol–disulfiram reaction.[12]

Polidocanol belongs to the class of detergent sclerosing solutions that are nonionic compounds. It consists of an apolar hydrophobic part (dodecyl alcohol) and a polar hydrophilic part (polyethylene-oxide chain) that is esterified. In solution, polidocanol is associated as macromolecules through electrostatic hydrogen bonding between the H^+ atom of the OH–group in one molecule, and the free electron-pair of an oxygen atom of a second molecule. This bonding results in the formation of a network. The sclerotherapeutic activity results from this double hydrophobic and hydrophilic action, and thus polidocanol is a 'detergent'.[12]

Polidocanol was introduced in 1936 as a local and topical anesthetic. Polidocanol has a noncyclic chemical structure. The anesthetic effect is not a direct function of its concentration but is optimum at a concentration between 3% and 4%. Polidocanol is unique among local anesthetics in its lack of an aromatic ring. As an aliphatic molecule, it is composed of a hydrophilic chain of polyethylene glycolic ether and a lipo-soluble radical of dodecylic alcohol.[3] It is used as a topical anesthetic agent in ointments and lotions for mucous membranes, including hemorrhoidal treatment.[12] It is also used as a local anesthetic for skin irritation, burns and insect bites and as an epidural anesthetic.[13-15]

Polidocanol is diluted in absolute alcohol and is available in 2-mL ampoules of 0.25%, 0.5%, 1%, 1.5%, 2%, 3% and 4%, as well as in 2-mL syringes at concentrations of 0.25%, 0.5% and 1%. Telangiectasias are treated with concentrations of 0.25% to 0.75%.[16] Varicose veins are treated with concentrations of 1% to 4%. A 4% solution is recommended for treatment of varicosities greater than 8 mm in diameter. A 3% solution is recommended for varicose veins 4 to 8 mm in diameter, 2% is recommended for varicose veins 2 to 4 mm in diameter, and 1% for veins 1 to 2 mm in diameter. The practitioner should take care not to exceed the maximum dose of polidocanol, which is 2 mg/kg per day. Polidocanol was approved by the FDA in March 2010.[3,17,18]

Advantages

- Effective at low concentrations
- Polidocanol is unique among sclerosing agents in that it is both painless to inject and does not produce cutaneous ulcerations, even with intradermal injection of concentrations less than 1.0%

- Can produce pigmentation but the degree of pigmentation produced may be less than that of other detergent sclerosing agents
- FDA approved

Disadvantages

- Allergic reactions though rare can occur
- Moderate risk for skin necrosis, pigmentation at high concentrations

Sodium Morrhuate

Sodium morrhuate is a mixture of sodium salts of the saturated and unsaturated fatty acids present in cod-liver oil. It is prepared by the saponification of selected cod-liver oils. Each milliliter contains morrhuate sodium, 50 mg; benzyl alcohol, 2% (as a local anesthetic); water for injection (as much as will suffice); and hydrochloric acid and/or sodium hydroxide to adjust the pH to approximately 9.5. It is available as a 5% concentration that can be diluted with normal saline (to the appropriate concentration) for the vessel to be treated. The FDA has approved the usage of sodium morrhuate for sclerosis of varicose veins.[3]

Advantage

- FDA approved

Disadvantages

- Extensive cutaneous necrosis and severe pain occurs when injected perivascularly
- Extremely caustic in nature
- Highest risk for anaphylaxis

Ethanolamine Oleate

Ethanolamine oleate is a synthetic mixture of ethanolamine and oleic acid with an empiric formula of $C_{20}H_{41}NO_3$. It is available as a 5% aqueous solution containing approximately 50 mg of ethanolamine oleate per milliliter. Benzyl alcohol, 2% by volume, is used as a preservative. The pH ranges from 8.0 to 9.0.

Early animal model studies suggest that ethanolamine completely inhibits coagulation at concentrations as low as 0.31%, and induces sclerosis via endothelial damage leading to fibrin-product deposition and thrombosis hours after exposure. Its excellent thrombosing effect adds to the efficacy of ethanolamine oleate sclerosis. The oleic acid component is responsible for the inflammatory action. Oleic acid may also activate coagulation in vitro by release of tissue factors and Hageman factor XII. The ethanolamine component suppresses fibrin clot formation. Prepared in 50 mg/mL of aqueous solution, it is available from its manufacturer in 2 mL ampoules. Standard dosing is usually one ampoule per session.[2,3] It is FDA approved for esophageal varices.

Advantages

- When compared to ethanol is its less severe and less-frequent side effects
- Ethanolamine does not invade the vascular wall as deeply as ethanol, reducing the potential risk to adjacent soft tissue structures and nerves

Disadvantages

- Even a 0.5% solution produces an unacceptable incidence of eschar, ulceration or pigmentation when injecting telangiectasias of less than 1 mm in diameter.
- Effect seen with extravascular administration is hemolysis with renal failure that requires prophylactic administration of albumin and treatment with haptoglobin.[19]
- Exacerbation of heart failure, pleural effusions and right sided heart failure has also been reported, likely related to the broad intravascular distribution of ethanolamine oleate.[19]

OSMOTIC SOLUTIONS

Hypertonic solutions, such as hypertonic saline, probably cause dehydration of endothelial cells through osmosis, causing endothelial destruction.[20] It is speculated that fibrin deposition with thrombus formation on the damaged vessel wall occurs through modification of the electrostatic charge of the endothelial cells.[21] For the vessel wall to be completely destroyed, the osmotic solution must be of sufficient concentration to diffuse throughout the entire vein wall. Hypertonic solutions have a predictable destructive power that is proportional to their osmotic concentration. Because dilution occurs with intravascular serum and blood, osmotic solutions have their greatest effect at or near the site of injection. In contrast, detergent sclerosing solutions can exert effective sclerosis for 5 to 10 cm along the course of the injected vessel.[3]

Hypertonic Saline

Hypertonic saline was first used to sclerose varicose veins by Linser[21] in 1926, and Kern and Angle[22] in 1929. With the advent of more effective, synthetic, detergent sclerosing solutions in the 1940s, its use declined. It is available in 23.4% and 11.7% concentrations; hypertonic saline is not an FDA-approved sclerosant but its use in sclerotherapy is off label. An extensive body of research in the dermatologic literature has demonstrated the safe and effective use of hypertonic saline for small, superficial venous structures such as telangiectasias, varicose veins and reticular veins.[23]

Use of special lighting, recumbent position of the patient, and repeated small injections have been used by practitioners to improve results and reduce potential side effects. Administration is from large central vessel to smaller peripheral vessels, and consistent postprocedural compression improves results. A key consideration is blood flow through a target vessel because mixing will reduce the effectiveness and control of the agent to the target tissues by blood flow movement. Therefore, there are significant limits to the vessel size that can be effectively targeted with hypertonic saline.[5,24]

Advantages

- Inexpensive, easy to store and concentrations can be easily adjusted by dilution
- There is no expected anaphylactic or allergic reaction when preservative-free preparations are used

Disadvantages

- Weak sclerosant
- The most common complication is residual blood pooling in treated vessels, which can be easily aspirated at follow up
- Nearby tissue necrosis including skin ulceration secondary to extravasation from the target vessel is the most concerning complication
- Painful to inject

Pain occurs during injection and skin discoloration may occur due to extravasated red blood cells. When extravasation occurs, massaging the injected tissue and removing any excess solution may achieve rapid diffusion of the hypertonic saline. Using lower concentrations of hypertonic saline may mitigate pain and skin discoloration.[25,26]

Because hypertonic saline diffuses to some extent through the blood vessel wall, nerves in the adventitia of the vein may be stimulated, causing pain. This diffusion may also lead to transient muscle cramping. Because osmotic agents are rapidly diluted in the bloodstream, they lose their potency within a short distance of injection. Thus, these agents are only rarely effective in treating veins larger than 3 to 4 mm in diameter.[3]

Modification of the Solution and the Technique

A number of modifications in injection technique have also been made to limit the pain of hypertonic saline. Bodian[27] found that muscle cramps occurring at the site of injection last 3 to 5 minutes, and are relieved with gentle massage or ambulation. To limit the risk of extravasation, he recommended injecting a small air bolus before injecting 0.5 to 1 mL of hypertonic saline; this ensures undiluted contact of the hypertonic saline with the intima to produce maximum irritation of the vessel. He believed that hemolysis caused by the sclerosing solution may lead to or exacerbate hemosiderin staining, and thus should be lessened by the prior injection of air, which washes out the RBCs from the vessel.[3]

Attempts have been made to reduce postinjection pain from hypertonic saline by the addition of local anesthetics such as lignocaine. However, this practice appears to be counterproductive because the local anesthetics are acidic (and therefore contribute to transient pain on injection) and have known allergenicity, the very properties that proponents of hypertonic saline wish to avoid. The addition of heparin to hypertonic saline in an attempt to prevent thrombosis in larger vessels and to reduce the incidence of thrombophlebitis and postsclerotherapy pigmentation has been found to be of no therapeutic benefit in treating telangiectasias.[1]

Hypertonic Glucose–Saline

Hypertonic saline (10%) and dextrose (25%) has been used as a sclerosing agent. A mixture of dextrose 250 mg/mL, sodium chloride 100 mg/mL, propylene glycol 100 mg/mL, and phenethyl alcohol 8 mg/mL (as a local anesthetic/preservative) at a pH of 5.9, is used for sclerosis of telangiectasias and small-diameter superficial varicosities.[28] It is essentially a hypertonic solution with a mechanism of action similar to hypertonic saline. The sodium chloride reinforces the sclerosing potency of dextrose according to some.

The maximum quantity to be injected during one visit is 10 mL in divided doses, with a 5-cm interval between each site of injection. (The maximum recommended amount to be injected at any one site is 1 mL.) The average dose per treated vein varies between 1 mL in the upper thigh and 0.1 mL in the lower leg.[3]

Advantages

- Less pain and local discomfort compared to hypertonic saline alone. Probably the decrease in osmolarity relative to 23.4% hypertonic saline that allows this combination to produce less pain and muscle cramping.
- Low risk of allergic reactions

Disadvantages

- Relatively weak sclerosing agent
- Not FDA approved for use as sclerosing agent

CHEMICAL IRRITANTS

Mechanism of Action

Chemical irritants also act directly on endothelial cells to produce endosclerosis. Chemical irritant sclerosing solution produces its end result of vascular fibrosis through the irreversible destruction of endothelial cells with resultant thrombus formation on the subendothelial layer.[3]

Chromated Glycerin/Glycerin

The most common sclerosant used worldwide for telangiectasias is a chemical class sclerosant called chromate glycerin. Reports, however, have surfaced regarding the efficacy of 72% glycerin which is an off-label FDA-approved drug. This agent is not commercially produced but can be obtained through compounding pharmacies. It is mixed with lidocaine with epinephrine, 1:10000 in a 2:1 ratio with a resultant concentration of 48% glycerin. The lidocaine minimizes pain with injection and decreases viscosity. The epinephrine helps with vessel constriction producing longer dwell times and helps with its chemical corrosive effect. Typically, tuberculin syringes are used for injection because of its viscosity. Injection should be slow to minimize injection pain and prevention of potential arteriolar crossover from high pressures delivered using tuberculin syringes. Slow injection is the rule for all sclerosants to minimize this side effect and the potential for vein matting.

Since glycerin is obtainable on formulary for use in cerebral edema and acute glaucoma, its availability makes it a promising alternative to more caustic sclerosing agents. The glycerin component is rapidly absorbed by the intestine and transformed into carbon dioxide or glycogen or is directly used for the synthesis of fatty acids.[29] Therefore, this solution must be used with caution in diabetic patients. The chromium alum component is a potent coagulating factor that increases the sclerosing power of glycerin. It also prevents the mild hematuria induced through the use of glycerin alone.[30,31]

Advantages

- Very low incidence of pigmentation, ulceration
- Very rare allergic reaction

Disadvantages

- Very weak sclerosant
- Has a high viscosity and local pain at injection (both of these drawbacks can be overcome partially by dilution with lidocaine)[3]
- Hematuria associated with ureteral colic can occur transiently after injection of large doses[3]

Ethanol

Ethanol is a sclerosing agent most commonly used for treating arteriovenous malformations. It kills cells by fixation, preserving cell morphology, and is thus listed as a 'chemical' sclerosing agent.[3] Its mechanism of action is a combination of cytotoxic damage induced by the denaturation and extraction of surface proteins, hypertonic dehydration of cells, and coagulation and thrombosis when blood products are present. All of these factors lead to fibrinoid necrosis.[32-34]

Ethanol's deep penetration into the vascular wall and lack of viscosity allows it to affect most tissues, although its reactions are not tissue specific.[19]

The effect is dependent on ethanol concentration, time of exposure and injection rate; rapid injection rates produce more endothelial damage and parenchymal necrosis with less thrombosis whereas slower rates produce more thrombosis, but less endothelial damage and necrosis.[35] Ethanol has broad applications in both vascular and nonvascular interventions, although its use is limited by high complication rates and morbidity. Dosing should not exceed 1 mL/kg, as studies have demonstrated systemic blood alcohol concentrations of up to 0.07% at this dose.[36] The use of ethanol in neurologically sensitive areas has decreased with the advent of more easily controlled polymers such as N-butyl cyanoacrylate (NBCA) and Onyx1.[2,37]

Advantages

- High response rate
- Cheap and easy to obtain
- Long shelf life
- Broad applications in vascular and nonvascular interventions

Disadvantages

- Alcohol intoxication—use with caution
- Very painful
- Skin necrosis and adjacent tissue damage
- Nerve impairment
- Hemoglobinuria
- Pulmonary artery hypertension
- Intoxication, bronchospasm, hyperthermia, cardiopulmonary collapse, death rarely[2,7]

Polyiodinated Iodine

It is a chemical irritant, dark brown in color with a strong sclerosing affect. It is composed of a stabilized water solution of iodide ions, sodium iodine and benzyl alcohol and used in concentrations of 0.2% to 12%.[3]

Advantage

- Strong sclerosant and allows treatment of largest veins

Disadvantages

- Pain on injection
- Necrosis of skin can occur
- Renal insufficiency
- Anaphylaxis (contraindicated in presence of hyperthyroidism and in patients with history of iodine allergy)[3,5]

OK 432

OK 432 is a biologic product created from the incubation of group A streptococcus with penicillin. Unlike other sclerotherapy agents, this agent is a natural killer cell activator and has been effectively used in the treatment of peritoneal carcinomatosis and pediatric lymphatic malformations by direct percutaneous injection.[35]

Bleomycin

Originally developed as an antibiotic and eventually used a chemotherapeutic agent due to its effect on DNA, bleomycin has been noted to cause fibrosis. This agent has been used for pleurodesis in the treatment of malignant pleural effusions. Bleomycin has had limited success in the treatment of pediatric lymphatic malformations, but has a good safety profile.[35]

Other agents used as sclerosants for various conditions like cysts include: N-butyl cyanoacrylate triamcinolone, doxycycline, tetracycline, acetic acid, phenol, pantopaque, bismuth, albendazole infusion and honey with variable results.[2]

SEQUENTIAL INJECTIONS OF DIFFERENT SCLEROSING SOLUTIONS

Sequential injections may be useful to enhance the efficacy of a milder sclerosing solution, either by increasing its potency or by the act of sequentially damaging endothelium. After mechanical trauma, endothelial cells are unable to generate various substances or to respond to circulating or locally produced substances.[38] In this damaged state, further injury may produce irreparable damage. In addition, combining a solution with another may produce an additive effect on its potency. Sodium tetradecyl sulfate 3% is currently the strongest sclerosant approved by the FDA. When treatment with this alone may prove ineffective, such as in patients with a large varicose vein or an area of high reflux, sequential use of hypertonic saline produces a stronger, synergistic effect. This technique has been reported recently using ultrasound guidance to sclerose the saphenofemoral junction.[3]

IDEAL SCLEROSANT

The ideal sclerosing solution should be painless on injection, free of all adverse effects, and would not produce allergic reactions and specific for damaged (varicose) veins. Although many agents have been used in treating varicose veins and telangiectasias, thus far none have completely satisfied the criteria for the ideal sclerosant.

Volumes, concentrations and progressive Dilution of Sclerosing Agents

A sclerosing reaction is induced by the contact of a sufficiently concentrated agent with the venous wall for a sufficient period of time. This adequate/effective concentration remains theoretical and ranges between a too strong, 'aggressive' concentration (responsible for transparietal burn and adverse reactions) and a too low, ineffective concentration (not inducing a sclerosing reaction). Contact should be even and homogeneous along the whole length of the vein being treated, and around the complete circumference of the vein. However, injection of liquid in a vein which is full of blood leads to some dilution, and in situ adequate concentrations are difficult to obtain. In veins smaller than 3 mm, a laminar flow of sclerosing agent replaces blood in the vein and no dilution occurs, but in bigger veins, a turbulence occurs and is responsible for dilution of the sclerosant.

The following is a method to compute theoretically how much sclerosing agent is necessary to fill up a vein. The inner volume V of a vein segment is: $V = L \times \pi \times (D/2)^2$, where L is the length, and D the inner diameter.[39]

Since volumes are proportional to the square of the radius, it is possible to inject a very long vein of small diameter with a small volume of liquid. When deciding the injected volume, the most important reference is the venous diameter.

The concentration of sclerosing agent decreases progressively when drifting away from the point of injection. Practically, when the liquid sclerosing agent is injected at a single point, the injected concentration is usually too high (in order to obtain a sufficiently long sclerosed zone, despite some dilution), and can induce side effects. To some extent, the problem can be addressed by injecting a greater volume of a milder solution or by injecting small volumes in multiple points close to each other. If a venous spasm occurs, or if some means allows a reduction in the vein diameter, the laminar flow will further improve the phenomenon. The ultimate evolution of this thinking is the use of foam, as described in a separate chapter.

An easy formula to develop a dilution chart for the various concentrations is (X mL) (stock solution %) = (desired total volume in mL) (desired concentration %).

Solve for *X* mL

This *X* volume is added to a volume of normal saline or sterile water to reach the desired total volume. This equation can be used to make the solution per syringe (3 mL and 10 mL) or in vials (10 mL and 30 mL) from which the solution can be aspirated.[5] The maximum dose and concentrations of sclerosing agents are given in Tables 6.2 and 6.3 respectively.

Finally, there is no known ideal sclerosant. Each has its advantages and disadvantages and thorough knowledge of the properties of each sclerosant, when applied with the fundamentals of good sclerotherapy practice will ensure optimum results.

Table 6.2: Maximum doses per session.[5]

Sclerosing agent	Maximum dose per session
Polidocanol	12 mL of 1% not to exceed 2 mg/kg
Sodium tetradecyl sulfate	10 mL of 3%
Hypertonic saline	8 mL of 23.4% (not more than 20 cc per session)
Sodium chloride solution with dextrose	10 mL
Glycerin 72% with lidocaine	15 mL plus (Final concentration glycerin 48%)

Table 6.3: Concentration of commonly used sclerosing agents.[40]

Vessel Size	Size	STS	POL
Telangiectasia	<1 mm	0.1–0.2	0.25-0.75
Venule	1–2 mm	0.2–0.4	0.5–1
Reticular vein	2–4 mm	0.2–0.4	2
Large varicose vein	>4 mm	0.4–0.75	3
Incompetent perforators		0.75–1	3
Vascular malformation		2–3	3
Figures are in percentage			

Table 6.4: Comparison of commonly used sclerosing agents.

Solution	Category	Advantages	Disadvantages	Vessels treated	Concentrations
Sodium tetradecyl sulfate	Detergent	Effective at low concentrations Less cytotoxic than ethanol Less painful/painless with intravascular injection Lower rates of systemic side effects FDA approved	Postsclerotherapy hyperpigmentation Epidermal necrosis with extravasation Allergic reactions	All sizes	0.1–0.2% telangiectasias, 0.2–0.4% reticular, 0.5–1.0% varicose, 1–3% axial varicose
Polidocanol	Detergent	Effective at low concentrations Painless Less pigmentation and necrosis FDA approved	Allergic reactions rarely	Small to medium	0.25–0.75% telangiectasias, 0.5–2.0% reticular, 1–3% varicose
Sodium morrhuate	Detergent	FDA approved	Extensive cutaneous necrosis and severe pain (when injected perivascularly) Extremely caustic in nature Highest risk for anaphylaxis	Small	Undiluted: telangiectasias Undiluted: reticular
Hypertonic sodium chloride solution	Osmotic agent	Inexpensive, easy to store concentrations can be easily adjusted Low allergenicity	Highly Painful injection High risk of skin necrosis, ulceration and pigmentation	Small	23.4–11.7% telangiectasias, 23.4% reticular

(Contd.)

Table 6.4: Comparison of commonly used sclerosing agents. (Contd.)

Solution	Category	Advantages	Disadvantages	Vessels treated	Concentrations
Ethanolamine oleate	Detergent	Less frequent and less severe side effects when compared to ethanol	Pain, ulceration, pigmentation Pulmonary complications Hemolytic reactions Acute renal failure Risk of urticaria and anaphylaxis		
Sodium chloride solution with dextrose	Osmotic agent	Low allergenicity Low risk of skin necrosis	Painful(less than hypertonic saline) Weak sclerosant	Small	Undiluted: telangiectasias Undiluted: reticular
Chromated glycerin	Chemical irritant	Less pigmentation and ulcerogenic potential	Very weak sclerosant Painful injection	Smallest	Undiluted to half strength: telangiectasias
Ethanol	Chemical irritant	High response rate Cheap and easy to obtain Long shelf life	Alcohol intoxication Very painful Skin necrosis Nerve impairment Hemoglobinuria Pulmonary artery hypertension Intoxication, bronchospasm, hyperthermia, cardiopulmonary collapse		Maximum dose of 1 mg/kg
Polyiodinated iodine	Chemical irritant	Strong sclerosant	Pain on injection Necrosis of skin Renal insufficiency Anaphylaxis	Largest	1–2% for up to 5 mm veins 2–6% for the largest veins

REFERENCES

1. Thibault PK. Sclerosing Agents. Available from: http://www.conferencematters.co.nz/pdf/ThibaultSCLEROSING%20AGENTS%20and%20their%20mechnism%20of%20action.pdf [Accessed on September 2017].
2. Albanese G, Kondo KL. Pharmacology of sclerotherapy. Semin Intervent Radiol. 2010;27(4):391-9.
3. Goldman MP, Weiss RA, Guex JJ. Mechanism of sclerotherapy. In: Goldman MP (Ed). Sclerotherapy: Treatment of Varicose and telangiectatic leg veins (5th edition). London: Elsevier Health Sciences; 2011. pp. 156-79.
4. Parsons ME. Sclerotherapy basics. Dermatol Clin. 2004;22:501-8.
5. Dietzek CL. Sclerotherapy: introduction to solutions and techniques. Perspectives in vascular surgery and endovascular therapy. 2007;19(3):317-24.
6. Saraf S. Role of sodium tetradecyl sulfate in venous malformations. Ind J Dermatol. 2006;51(4):258.
7. Sacchidanand S, Nagesh TS. Sclerotherapy. In: Venkataram M (Ed). ACS (I) Textbook on Cutaneous and Aesthetic Surgery (1st edition). New Delhi: Jaypee Medical Publishers; 2012. pp. 452-62.
8. Reiner L. The activity of anionic surface active compounds in producing vascular obliteration. Proc Soc Exp Bio Med. 1946;62:49-54.
9. Fegan WG. Continuous compression technique of injecting varicose veins. Lancet. 1963;2(7299):109-12.
10. Gomes AS. Embolization therapy of congenital arteriovenous malformations: use of alternate approaches. Radiology. 1994;190(1):191-8.
11. Ajekigbe L, Stothard J. The effectiveness of sodium tetradecyl sodium in the treatment of wrist ganglia. Can J Plast Surg. 2006;14(1):28-30.
12. Schulz KH. [The use of allylpoly-ethyleneoxide derivatives as surface anesthetics]. Dermatol Wochenschr. 1952;126(28):657-62.
13. Soehring K, Scriba K, Frahm M, et al. [On the pharmacology of alkylpolyethylene oxide derivatives. I. Studies on acute and subchronic toxicity in various animals]. Arch Int Pharmacodyn Ther. 1951;87(3):301-20.
14. Siems KJ, Soehring K. [Blockage of sensory nerves by perdural and paravertebral injection of alcylpolyethylenoxide ethers in guinea pigs]. Arzneimittelforschung. 1952;2(3):109-11.
15. Olesch B. Neuere Erkenntisse zur Pharmakokinetik von polidocanol (Aethoxysklerol). Vasomed Aktuell. 1990;4:22.
16. Carlin MC, Ratz JL. Treatment of telangiectasia: comparison of sclerosing agents. J Dermatol Surg Oncol. 1987;13(11):1181-6.
17. Fronek H. Fundamentals of Phlebology: Venous Disease for Clinicians. Royal Society of Medicine Press; 2007.
18. Feied CF. Sclerosing Solutions. The Vein Book. New York: Elsevier; 2007. pp. 125-38.
19. Hyodoh H, Hori M, Akiba H, et al. Peripheral Vascular Malformations: Imaging, Treatment Approaches, and Therapeutic Issues. Radiographics. 2005;25(Suppl 1): S159-71.
20. Cacciola E, Giustolisi R, Musso R, et al. Activation of contact phase of blood coagulation can be induced by the sclerosing agent polidocanol: possible additional mechanism of adverse reaction during sclerotherapy. J Lab Clin Med. 1987;109(2):225-6.
21. Imhoff E, Stemmer R. Classification and mechanism of action of sclerosing agents. Phlebologie. 1969;22(2):145.

22. Kern HM, Angle LW. The chemical obliteration of varicose veins: a clinical and experimental study. J Am Med Assoc. 1929;93(8):595-601.
23. Goldman MP. A comparison of sclerosing agents: clinical and histologic effects of intravascular sodium morrhuate, ethanolamine oleate, hypertonic saline (11.7%), and sclerodex in the dorsal rabbit ear vein. J Dermatol Surg Oncol. 1991; 17(4):354-62.
24. Tisi PV, Beverley C, Rees A. Injection sclerotherapy for varicose veins. Cochrane Database Syst Rev. 2006;18(4):CD001732.
25. Abrams HL. Abrams' angiography: interventional radiology. In: Baum S, Pentecost MJ (Eds). Abrams' Angiography: Interventional Radiology. Philadelphia: Lippincott Williams & Wilkins; 2006.
26. Sadick NS. Hyperosmolar versus detergent sclerosing agents in sclerotherapy. J Dermatol Surg Oncol. 1994;20(5):313-6.
27. Bodian EL. Sclerotherapy. Semin Dermatol. 1987;6(3):238-48.
28. Mantse L. A mild sclerosing agent for telangiectasias. J Dermatol Surg Oncol. 1985;11(9):855.
29. Martindale W. The Extra Pharmacopoeia (28th edition). London: Pharmaceutical Press; 1982.
30. Jausion H. Glycérine chromée et sclérose des ectasies veineuses. Masson; 1933.
31. Jausion H, Medioni G, Pecker A, et al. La sclerose des varices et des hemorrhoids par le glycerine chromee. Bull Memoires Soc Med Hospitaux Paris. 1932;587.
32. Ellman BA, Green CE, Eigenbrodt E, et al. Renal infarction with absolute ethanol. Investigat Radiol. 1980;15(4):318-22.
33. Do YS, Yakes WF, Shin SW, et al. Ethanol embolization of arteriovenous malformations: interim results. Radiology. 2005;235(2):674-82.
34. Mourao GS, Hodes JE, Gobin YP, et al. Curative treatment of scalp arteriovenous fistulas by direct puncture and embolization with absolute alcohol: report of three cases. J Neurosurg. 1991;75(4):634-7.
35. Dubois J, Garel L, Gordon Culham JA. Pediatric interventional angiography. In: Baum S, Pentecost MJ (Eds). Abrams' Angiography Interventional Radiology (2nd edition). Philadelphia: Lippincott Williams and Wilkins; 2006. pp. 1047-68.
36. Becker GH, Holden RW, Heun YY, et al. Ablation with absolute alcohol. In: Castaneda-Zuniga WR, Tadavarthy SM (Eds). Interventional Radiology. Baltimore: Williams and Wilkins; 1992. pp. 135-52.
37. Steiner F, FitzJohn T, Tan ST. Ethanol sclerotherapy for venous malformation. ANZ J Surg. 2016;86(10):790-5.
38. Vanhoutte PM. The endothelium—modulator of vascular smooth-muscle tone. N Engl J Med. 1988;319(8):512-3.
39. Hoeffner U, Vanhoutte PM. Endothelial factors and regulation of vascular tone. In: Vanhoutte PM (Ed). Return Circulation and Norepinephrine: An Update. Paris: John Libbey Eurotext; 1991. pp. 15-30.
40. Khunger N, Sacchidanand S. Standard guidelines for care: sclerotherapy in dermatology. Indian J Dermatol Venereol Leprol. 2011;77(2):222-31.

CHAPTER 7

Sclerotherapy for Varicose Veins

Nagesh TS, Sacchidanand S, Dinker Belle Rai

INTRODUCTION

Sclerotherapy is the targeted chemical ablation of varicose veins by intravenous injection of a liquid or foamed sclerosing drug.[1] The extent of damage to the blood vessel wall determines the effectiveness of the solution. Sclerotherapy has been extensively used by dermatosurgeons in the management of superficial varicose veins and other venous abnormalities.[2,3]

HISTORY

Earlier reports mention the use of a slender rod of iron by Hippocrates. In 1840s, Monteggio and Leroy D'Etoilles have tried absolute alcohol, and later in 1851, ferric chloride was used by Charles Gabriel Pravaz.[4] Injection of irritant substances into the vein for purpose of obliteration has been frequently mentioned in the French literature of last century. Strong caustic and toxic substances were used for injections. Iodine was used as a sclerosant by Beniamino Schiassi in 1908. Linser started the use of 20% sodium chloride solution. Sodium salicylate in a concentration of 20–40% solution was used by Sicard and his colleagues. Nobl has tried injections of 50% dextrose, and a mixture containing equal parts of dextrose and levulose with 4% sucrose. 25% sodium salicylate and 10% sodium chloride was used by Meisen.[5]

Objectives and Mechanism of Sclerotherapy

Varicose vein is one of the clinical manifestations of venous hypertension. Around 17 to 50% of people with varicose veins have skin findings. Chronic venous insufficiency (CVI) and superficial venous insufficiency can be treated by sclerotherapy or surgical treatment of the superficial venous system.[6] The ultimate goal of any interventional procedure is to normalize venous physiology.

The efficacy of calf muscle pump increases with treatment of incompetent perforators and varicose veins by sclerotherapy, resulting in an improved clearance of extravascular fluid.[6] Venous ulcers and stasis eczema also heal faster after undergoing sclerotherapy.[7] The irreversible endothelial cellular damage and exposure of underlying subendothelial layer in a dose-dependent manner after sclerotherapy leads to vascular fibrosis and obliteration. The response to sclerotherapy depends on the concentration of sclerosant. Too weak, a sclerosant will not cause any endothelial injury; if little stronger, will damage the vessel but recanalization occurs forming an incompetent pathway; and if too strong, can flow to adjacent vessels causing extensive tissue necrosis. Injection of an appropriate amount of sclerosant in appropriate concentrations which causes irreversible damage to the endothelium of the abnormal vessel, without damaging the normal vessels is the key to successful outcome from sclerotherapy.[4] Injection of the sclerosant and its subsequent dilution with blood results in three zones. Zone 1 is the site of irreversible endothelial injury which scleroses completely and is replaced by fibrous tissue. Partial or complete thrombosis of the vessel takes place in zone 2 which eventually recanalizes. In zone 3, the sclerosant is diluted to below its injurious concentration, without causing any endothelial injury.[4] The concentration of sclerosant used, vessel diameter and the position of the patient determines the extent of different zones.

The objectives of sclerotherapy include:[1,8]
- Ablation of varicose veins
- Prevention and treatment of complications of chronic venous disorders (CVD)
- Improvement and/or relief of venous symptoms
- Improvement of quality of life
- Improvement of venous function
- Improvement of the aesthetic appearance

INDICATIONS OF SCLEROTHERAPY IN VARICOSE VEINS[1,8,9]

- Pain
- Incompetent saphenous veins
- Major tributaries of greater and lesser saphenous veins
- Incompetent perforating veins
- Lateral venous system varicosities, reticular varicose veins
- Residual and recurrent varicose veins after surgery
- Complications of varicose veins like stasis dermatitis and venous ulcers
- Cosmetic—telangiectasias/spider webs

CONTRAINDICATIONS[1,7-9]

Absolute Contraindications

- Acute superficial or deep vein thrombosis
- Local infection in the area of sclerotherapy or severe generalized infection

- Immobility, confinement to bed
- Advanced peripheral arterial occlusive disease (stage 3 or 4)
- Hyperthyroidism (in the case of sclerosants containing iodine)
- Pregnancy in the first trimester and after the 36th week of gestation
- Known allergy to the sclerosant
- Severe systemic disease

Relative Contraindications

- Leg edema
- Saphenofemoral junction incompetence
- Thrombophilia with history of deep vein thrombosis
- Long-standing diabetes
- Peripheral arterial occlusive disease stage II
- Poor general health
- Myocardial decompensation
- Migraine
- Bronchial asthma
- Marked allergic diathesis
- Known hypercoagulability

SCLEROSING SOLUTIONS[8,9,10]

There are various sclerosing solutions available. The parameters to be considered in selecting a sclerosant include the diameter of the vessel to be treated, reflux, previous treatment response, minimal sclerosing concentration, pain tolerance and the complications associated with the sclerosant.

Sclerosing solutions are classified into three groups, based on their mechanisms of destruction of the endothelium; detergent agents, osmotic agents and chemical irritants. The details of different sclerosants will be discussed in the chapter 6 on sclerosing solutions.

Consent before Sclerotherapy

The patients should be informed about the various aspects of sclerotherapy, its effectiveness and complications associated with the procedure. Patients should be informed about:
- Various treatment options with their advantages and disadvantages
- Procedure of sclerotherapy and the post-treatment management
- Frequently occurring adverse events and serious risks
- Treatment outcome, success rate and recurrence rate
- Follow-up needed

PRE-PROCEDURE ASSESSMENT[1,11]

Case Selection

Any treatment aimed at an individual with varicose veins should consider the likely benefits of a particular intervention in three areas:
1. Cosmetic benefit
2. Symptomatic benefit
3. Prevention of progression of venous insufficiency and venous ulceration

The correlation between symptoms and severity of varicose veins is so poor that it is very difficult to predict the likely outcome after intervention as far as symptoms are concerned. As a general observation, patients who obtain benefit from properly fitted graduated elastic hosiery are likely to benefit from intervention in appropriate cases. If the procedure is in a patient who has already developed signs of CVI, positive outcome is assured. If the purpose of the intervention is cosmetic, it is reasonable to go ahead after careful discussion with the patients about the risks and benefits, as with any other cosmetic procedure.

A detailed evaluation of patient with varicose veins has been discussed in the earlier chapter. A detailed history including general medical condition, a thorough clinical evaluation and venous doppler is very important before taking the patient for sclerotherapy.

Examination

Physical examination to assess the skin for evidence of stasis dermatitis, stasis ulcer, examination of the venous system for varicosity, small vessels and large vessels and status of perforators is essential. Examination should include looking for evidence of previous deep vein thrombosis. Arterial pulses should be checked properly.

Procedure

Materials Required[12] (Fig. 7.1)

- Cotton balls soaked in spirit
- Protective gloves
- Disposable syringes of 1 cc or 3 cc with 30 gauge disposable transparent hub needles
- Elastocrepe for compression
- Hypoallergenic tape
- Topical nitroglycerine ointment (2%)
- Sclerosing solutions (stored separately from injectable) diluted with normal saline
- Magnifying loupes or lenses

Sclerotherapy for Varicose Veins

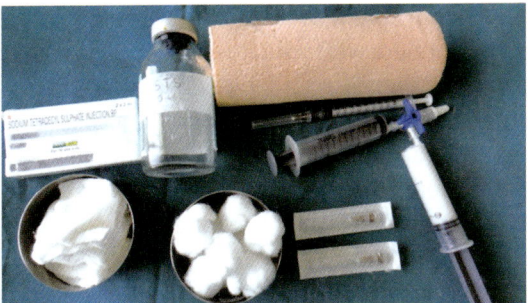

Fig. 7.1: Sclerotherapy tray.

Table 7.1: Indications for different concentrations.

Higher concentration	Lower concentration
• Younger patients • Thick walled vessels (use palpation) • Hand/feet/pretibial veins • Vessels >4 mm in diameter to compensate for dilution	• Age >60 years • 0.6–0.9 mm in diameter elevated spider veins • Thin walled vessels • Easy bruisability • History of spontaneous bleeding following minor trauma

SCLEROSANT CONCENTRATIONS[13]

Indications for lower and higher concentrations are shown in Table 7.1.

PRINCIPLES OF VARICOSE VEIN SCLEROTHERAPY[6]

The important steps to be considered while performing sclerotherapy for varicose veins are:
- Proximal to distal injection
- Larger vein to be treated before smaller veins
- Vein must be emptied of blood by various maneuvers
- Direct finger pressure should be applied in spreading and compressing motion after injection
- Reflux points should be determined initially and treated specifically
- Immediate and adequate compression is important
- Adequate ambulation should be recommended immediately after treatment.

PATIENT PREPARATION[12]

A comfortable position for the patient and doctor with proper lighting is very important for performing sclerotherapy. The patient should be in recumbent position that allows convenient access to the veins to be treated. Motorized table with height adjustment will facilitate easy access to all regions of the legs. The area to be treated is exposed adequately and cleaned thoroughly with spirit or povidone-iodine. Usually anesthesia, intralesional or topical, is not required. An anxious patient is counselled, and an analgesic or antianxiety drug may be administered. The sclerosant is diluted to the required concentration (Table 7.2) with distilled water or saline and loaded in a syringe.

TECHNIQUES

Techniques depend on the size of veins as follows.

Sclerotherapy Techniques for Large Veins[6]

There are two common techniques employed: (1) Fegan's technique and (2) Sigg's technique.[6]

Fegan's Technique

This technique is commonly used with minor modifications. The patient is asked to sit with the leg in dependent position. The varicose vein is cannulated with a needle or angiocatheter. Followed by this, leg is elevated to allow drainage of blood. A small amount of blood is withdrawn into the syringe to ensure the placement of needle in the varicose veins. Too much blood may cause dilution of the sclerosant. Approximately 0.5–1 mL of sclerosant is slowly injected along with application of finger pressure several centimeters above and below the injection site. This increases the effectiveness of the procedure and also confines the action of the sclerosing solution to the affected site. Finger pressure is continued for 30–60 seconds followed by immediate application of compression with a foam pad. An elastic tape or bandage is applied to maintain compression adequately. This method is used for large veins and also for incompetent perforators.

Table 7.2: Concentration of sclerosants depending on the vessel size.

Sclerosing solution	Vessels treated	Concentrations
Sodium tetradecyl sulfate	All sizes	0.1–0.2% telangiectasias 0.2–0.5% reticular 0.5–1.0% varicose 1.0–3.0% axial varicose
Polidocanol	Small to medium	0.25–0.5% telangiectasias 0.5–1.0% reticular 1.0–3.0% varicose

Note: Concentration used will be less when using foam sclerotherapy for the same diameter vessel.

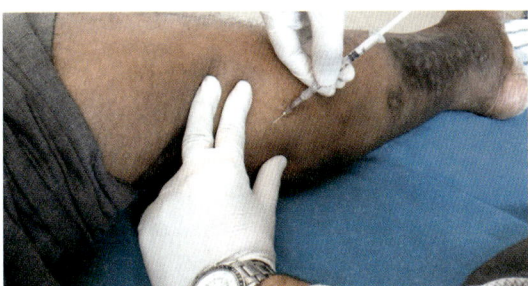

Fig. 7.2: Position of hand while injecting.

The perforators can be marked during venous Doppler study. The site of needle entry is at the fascial defects through which perforator course can be palpated.

Variation of Fegan's technique: The varicosities are marked with the patient in standing position and the injection is in recumbent or slight reverse Trendelenburg position. Movement of leg and chances of displacement of needle can be minimized with this method. After the injection the leg is elevated and compression is applied. Cannulation is usually easy as the varicosities are marked and patient is in supine position. Finger pressure and outward movement from the injection site helps not only in spreading the sclerosant but also to promote contact with greater surface area of the varicosity by emptying the vessel (Fig. 7.2).

Sigg's Technique

This method using an open needle was commonly used for sclerosing saphenous junctions. A needle without the syringe attached is inserted and manipulated till the blood drips followed by injection of the sclerosant.

Sclerotherapy for Reticular Veins (Figs. 7.3 to 7.6)

The technique of injection of reticular veins is similar to large veins, however the concentration and volume of sclerosing solution is reduced.[6] All sources of reflux has to be treated either by surgery or sclerotherapy before injecting the reticular veins. The reticular veins are superficial and blue. Injections can be made with patient in recumbent position. A 3 mL syringe with a 30 gauge needle is used. On feeling the sensation of piercing the vein, small amount of blood is withdrawn to confirm the proper placement of needle. Around 0.5 mL of the sclerosant is slowly injected. The sclerosant solution commonly used are sodium tetradecyl sulfate (STS) and polidocanol. Multiple sittings are needed with a treatment interval of 4–8 weeks between each session.

70 Sclerotherapy in Dermatology

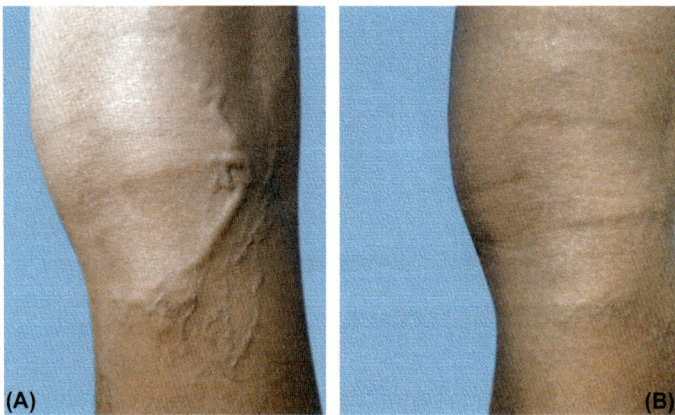

Figs. 7.3A and B

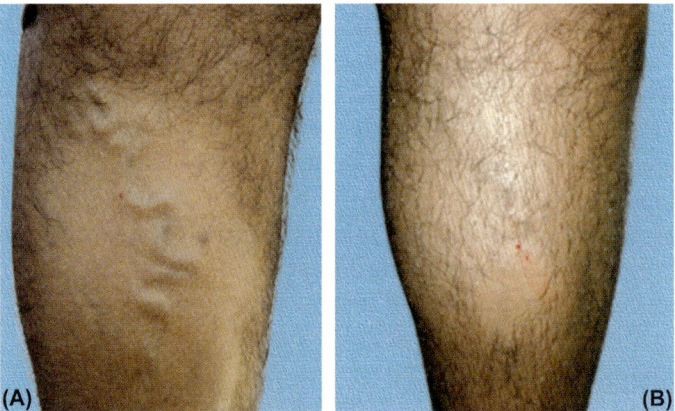

Figs. 7.4A and B

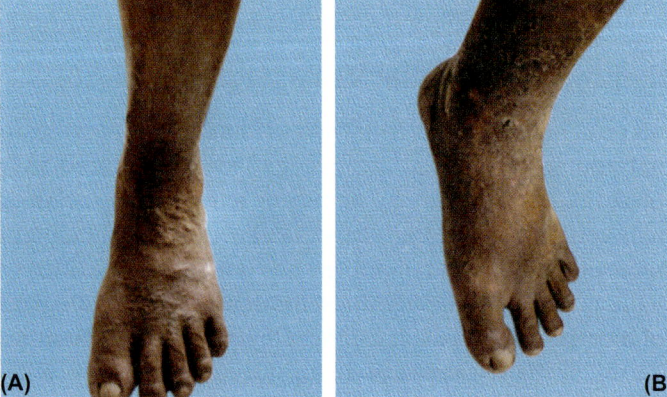

Figs. 7.5A and B

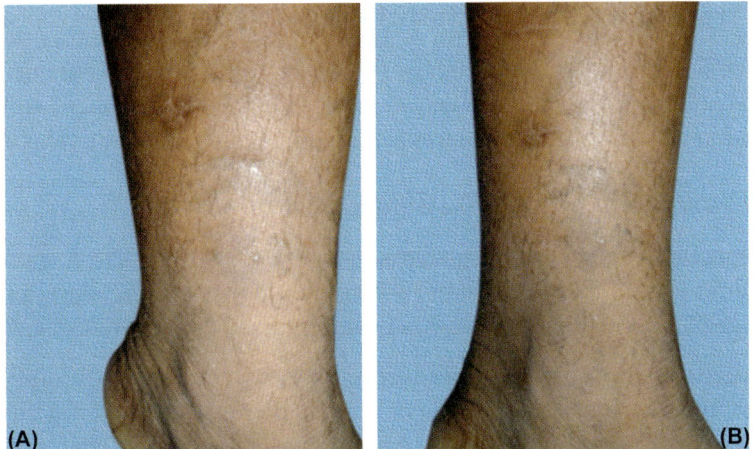

Figs. 7.6A and B: Before and after sclerotherapy for the small veins.

Sclerotherapy for Telangiectasia

Microsclerotherapy of telangiectasias using extremely fine needle was developed and popularized by Biegelson. Morrhuate sodium was used by him, which caused various complications like pigmentation, necrosis and allergic reaction. Hypertonic saline with or without heparin, and STS were used later which showed few adverse effects with good results.[14]

Microsclerotherapy can be done for any small telangiectatic vessel or venule on the skin. Superficial linear or radiating vessels on the lower extremities show a good response. Telangiectasias on the face and bright red telangiectasias on the legs which have a rapid refilling time are less responsive to sclerotherapy and tend to recur after treatment. Also there are chances of cutaneous necrosis if the sclerosant reaches the arteriolar feeding loop.[15]

Photographic documentation is important before the procedure. Moisturizing creams should be avoided on the day of procedure as it can cause slipperiness of the skin.

The procedure is performed with the patient in supine position. Reticular veins and telangiectasias can be best visualized in sunlight or fluorescent lighting.

Most telangiectasias are in the upper dermis. The needle has to enter almost parallel to the skin surface; the needle can be bent with the bevel up. If the needle is outside the vessel, there will be an immediate superficial wheal. A gentle upward traction while advancing the needle can ensure superficial placement. The advantage of injecting with bevel up is that it reduces the chances of transaction of the vessel.[14]

Ultrasound Guided Sclerotherapy

Ultrasound guided sclerotherapy (UGS) for the superficial venous system was published in 1989.[16] Initially it was used to treat incompetent saphenous axes and later in 1992, it was used for incompetent perforating veins also.[17]

Techniques of Ultrasound Guided Sclerotherapy

Generally, strong sclerosing solutions are used in UGS. STS is more commonly used. Foam sclerosants are commonly used these days for UGS[18] (Fig. 7.7). Foam sclerotherapy has been discussed in a separate chapter.

Patient positioning: The procedure is done with the patients in supine positon. The leg to be treated should be level, and externally rotated at the hip for injection of veins on the medial aspect of the leg. The knee is slightly flexed in order to relax all muscle groups. For small incompetent veins, semi-reclining position will dilate the veins slightly, thereby helps in ultrasound visualization and subsequent injection. Prone position with the foot supported by a pillow will help in the treatment of veins on the posterior thigh or calf.[18] This is important when injection of the short saphenous vein near the popliteal fossa; where the veins will be compressed if the knee is totally extended.

Technique: The most commonly used method is the closed needle technique.[19] In this technique, the needle is attached to the syringe containing the sclerosant at all times. The procedure may be performed with the assistance of a radiologist or with the treating doctor performing both the ultrasound and the injections alone.[19]

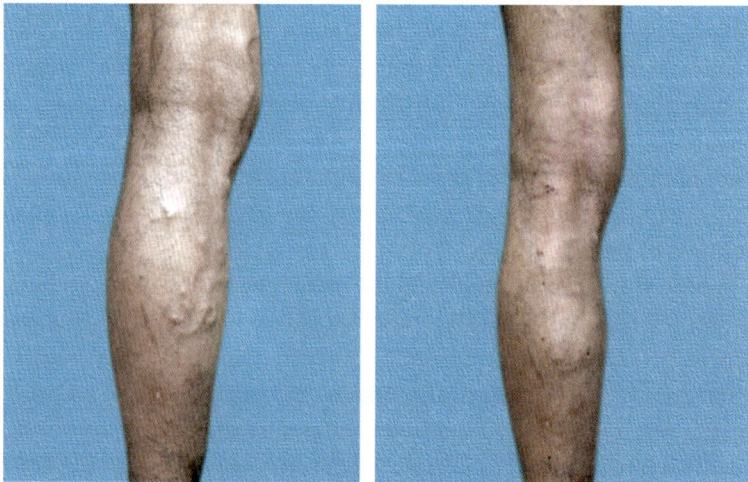

Fig. 7.7: Before and after ultrasound guided sclerotherapy.

Source: Dhanraj Chavan, KIMS (Krishna Institute of Medical Sciences, Karad), Satara, Maharashtra, India.

The proximal origin of the venous reflux is treated first. The site of the vein to be injected will be localized in transverse view by the radiologist.[20] The depth of the vein below the skin surface will be noted which will determine the angle of approach of the needle. Then the injection can be performed either with the vein viewed in transverse section, or in sagittal or longitudinal section. Both approaches can be used depending on the technical variables associated with each individual injection.[19] It is easier to cannulate the vein with the transverse approach. It is therefore particularly useful when injecting smaller veins less than 3 mm in diameter. In the longitudinal approach, the direction of flow of the sclerosant can be observed and the linear array probes can be used to compress the segment of vein for a length of about 50 mm during the injection, thereby allowing better contact of the sclerosant with the vein wall at the injection site.

The imaging frequency of the transducer used varies from 7.5 MHz to 15 MHz.[18] More superficial veins are better visualized with higher frequencies, and deeper subcutaneous veins with the lower frequencies. Most transducers will have an indicator liner or LED that will indicate the alignment of the sagittal plane of the transducer. When the needle pierces the skin, the tip should be visualized by the ultrasound. Adequate amounts of ultrasound gel need to be applied to the skin to obtain optimum visualization.[18]

An indentation will be seen on the vein wall once the needle tip makes contact with the target vein. At this stage, vein wall is pierced, and after this, the needle can be seen within the lumen and a small amount of blood is drawn into the needle hub to confirm correct intraluminal positioning of the needle tip. A small volume of sclerosant should be injected to look for the ultrasound image to be flowing into the vein. Extravasation is readily visible on the B-mode image and is manifested as a separation between the vein wall and the perivenous tissues. When the initial small volume is seen to flow intraluminally, the remainder of the injection is then completed under continuous ultrasound imaging.[18]

SUMMARY

Sclerotherapy is a simple and effective procedure for the treatment of varicose veins. Even the larger veins can also be treated effectively with UGS. Also sclerotherapy can be used for cosmetic indications like telangiectasias. The sequelae of varicose veins can be prevented if varicose veins are treated in the initial stages. Sclerotherapy can be done as an outpatient procedure, and hence is associated with very minimal morbidity, mortality and loss of work time compared to surgery. Sclerotherapy has emerged as a simple, safe and effective treatment modality for management of venous abnormalities, both therapeutically and esthetically. The introduction of foam sclerotherapy has carried the field further forward. New advances in laser ablation have opened new avenues for management of these common therapeutic and aesthetic problems.

REFERENCES

1. Rabe E, Breu FX, Cavezzi A, et al. European guidelines for sclerotherapy in chronic venous disorders. Phlebology. 2014;29:338-54.
2. Goldman MP. Treatment of varicose and telangiectatic leg veins: double-blind prospective comparative trial between aethoxyskerol and sotradecol. Dermatol Surg. 2002;28:52-5.
3. Lorenz MB, Gkogkolou P, Goerge T. Sclerotherapy of vacose veins in dermatology. J Dtsch Dermatol Ges 2014;12(5):391-3.
4. Feied C. Sclerosing solutions. In: Bergan JJ (Ed). The Vein Book. USA: Elsevier Academic Press; 2007. pp. 125-31.
5. De Takas G. Varicose veins and their sequelae. JAMA. 1929;92:775-9.
6. Goldman MP, Weiss RA, Bergan JJ. Diagnosis and treatment of varicose veins: a review. J Am Acad Dermatol. 1994;31:393-413.
7. Subbarao NT, Aradhya SS, Veerabhadrappa NH. Sclerotherapy in the management of varicose veins and its dermatological complications. Ind J Dermatol Venereol Leprol. 2013;79:383-8.
8. Weiss MA, Hsu JT, Neuhaus I, et al. Consensus for sclerotherapy. Dermatol Surg. 2014;40(12):1309-18.
9. Weiss RA, Weiss MA. Treatment of varicose and telangiectatic veins. In: Freedberg JM, Eisen AZ, Wolff K, et al. (Eds). Fitzpatrick's Dermatology in General Medicine (6th edition). USA: McGraw Hill Publishers; 2003. pp. 2549-56.
10. Sadick N, Li C. Small vessel sclerotherapy. Dermatol Clin. 2001;19:475-81.
11. Khunger N, Sacchidanand S. Standard guidelines for care: sclerotherapy in dermatology. Ind J Dermatol Venereol Leprol. 2011;77:222-30.
12. Weiss RA, Weiss MA. Sclerotherapy treatment of telangiectasias. In: Bergan JJ (Ed). The Vein Book. USA: Elsevier Academic Press; 2007. pp. 133-8.
13. Duffy DM. Sclerotherapy. In: Dover JS, Alam M, Nguyen TH, (Eds). Treatment of Leg Veins. USA: Elsevier Saunders; 2006. pp. 71-105.
14. Goldman MP, Guex JJ, Weiss RA. Clinical methods for sclerotherapy of Telangiectasias. In: Goldman MP, Guex JJ, Weiss RA (Eds). Sclerotherapy: Treatment of Varicose and Telangiectatic Leg Veins (5th edition). USA: Elsevier Saunders Publications; 2011. pp. 315-35.
15. Goldman MP, Weiss RA, Brody HJ, et al. Treatment of facial telangiectasia with sclerotherapy, laser surgery, and/or electrodessication: a review. J Dermatol Surg Oncol. 1993;19:899.
16. Knight RM, Vin F, Zygmunt JA. Ultrasonic guidance of injections into the superficial venous system. In: Davy A, Stemmer R (eds). Phlebologie' 89. Montrouge, France: John Libbey Eurotext Ltd; 1989.
17. Thibault PK, Lewis WA. Recurrent varicose veins. Part 2: injection of incompetent perforating veins using ultrasound guidance. J Dermatol Surg Oncol. 1992; 18:895-900.
18. Thibault P. Sclerotherapy and ultrasound guided sclerotherapy. In: Bergan JJ (Ed). The Vein Book. USA: Elsevier Academic Press; 2007;189-99.
19. Varcoe PF. Ultrasound guided sclerotherapy: efficacy, adverse events and dosing: an international survey. ANZ J Phleb. 2003;7:17-24.
20. Kanterr A, Thibault P. Saphenofemoral junction incompetence treated by ultrasound guided sclerotherapy. Dermatol Surg. 1996;22(7):648-52.

CHAPTER 8

Foam Sclerotherapy

Savitha AS, Sujala S

INTRODUCTION

Foam sclerotherapy has become widely used in recent years and has been found that the medium-term outcome is similar to that of surgery in varicose veins management.[1] It has been shown that foam sclerosants are more effective than the same volume of liquid sclerosant of similar strength.[2] Peroperative foam sclerotherapy (PFS) has been used to complete the more invasive parts of the surgical procedures.[3]

HISTORY

Foote described a method of foam sclerotherapy in 1944.[4] This was improved by Orbach in 1950, wherein he published a paper describing the use of a foam which he created by vigorously shaking a syringe containing air and sclerosant to produce a froth.[5] In 1995 Cabrera et al. suggested that foam could be created using carbon dioxide mixed with polidocanol (POL), a detergent sclerosant. Cabrera used sclerotherapy with foam, guiding his injections by ultrasound imaging. He called his invention 'microfoam', comprising very small bubbles in contrast to the large bubble froths that had been used previously.[6]

METHODS OF FOAM PREPARATION

Currently there are three main options of foam preparation:
1. High-speed beating in a carbon dioxide-rich atmosphere—Cabrera's technique[6]
2. Specific gas mixture combined with polidocanol and passed through a patented sieve in an aerosol canister.[7]
3. *Tessari method:* The Tessari technique is characterized by the generation of foam by turbulent mixture of fluid and air in two syringes connected via a three-way stopcock.
    a. Two syringes, one loaded with a volume of room air and the other with a volume of detergent sclerosant, polidocanol or sodium tetradecyl sulfate are connected via three way stopcock. The mixing ratio for sclerosant:air is 1:4 to 1:5[8] (Fig. 8.1).

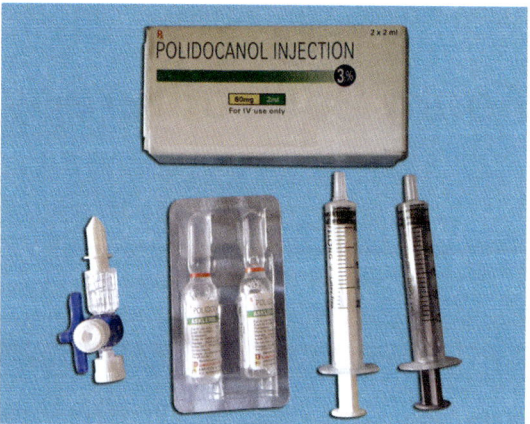

Fig. 8.1: Polidocanol foam prepared using Tessari method.

b. The air solution mix is passed quickly 10 to 20 times between the two syringes, which allows for rapid agitation and foam creation.[8] The aperture of the three-way stopcock can be made smaller if rotated off center creating a thicker, longer lasting foamed state.

c. Modifications of Tessari:
- Two-way female connector[2]
- Automated foaming device Turbofoam (Kreussler Pharma, France)[7]

4. *Monfreux technique*: It is characterized by the generation of negative pressure by drawing back the plunger in a glass syringe whose tip is tightly closed. The resulting air inlet generates a large bubbled, rather fluid foam.[9]

FOAM STABILITY

Foam stability is affected by foam composition, foam volume and injection technique.[10] Homogeneity of bubble size, viscosity and temperature, all influence the quality and longevity of foam. Heat increases the stability of foam.[11] Bubble size is inversely related to the difference in density between a liquid and gas, as represented in the equation below:[12]

$$d_p = \left(\frac{6 d_o \sigma}{\Delta \rho g} \right)^{1/3}$$

Where,
d_p = bubble diameter
d_o = orifice diameter
σ = surface tension
$\Delta \rho$ = difference in density between a liquid and gas.

Carbon dioxide is 1.5 times denser than room air; therefore, foam bubbles prepared from carbon dioxide are smaller than those of air. Foam bubbles produced via Tessari technique are smaller (less than 100 μm) in size as compared to the larger bubbles produced in the Monfreux technique. This smaller bubble size is associated with an increased surface area of sclerosant, increased displacement of blood inside the vessel, and decreased likelihood of mixing with blood following the initial injection. Therefore, an increased amount of sclerosant can be delivered to the endothelial cells.[13,14] Carbon dioxide has a greater diffusibility into blood than nitrogen (dominant in room air), resulting in reduced half-life for carbon dioxide foam. A mixture of 70% CO_2 and 30% O_2 can be used to make foam, increasing the half-life. Pure CO_2 makes short lived, poor quality foam.[15]

Room air foam half-life depends on the percent of sclerosant used. Around 1% concentration of STS and POL has a half-life of 90–120 s respectively.[16] However half-life of carbon dioxide foam does not depend on the sclerosant concentration.

Silicone coating present in syringes and connectors has antifoaming properties. Though studies by Rao et al. have shown that the amount of silicone in syringes does not affect foam stability, variations have been found between different syringe companies due to variations in silicone content.[16,17]

Before injection, small bubbles in foam tend to unite as bigger units (Laplace's law) and in sometime the foam gets replaced by larger bubbles whose effect will be observed with Orbach's air block.[7] Stability of foam should not be tested on foam created 90 s in advance. The preparation of foam does not change the concentration of sclerosing agent. Typically foam lasts 60–120 s before it breaks down. As the foam dissipates in the injecting syringe, it can be recreated in the same fashion as outlined above in Tessari method. A 5 μm intravenous filter can be inserted between the syringes to improve the quality of foam and increase the foam stability by 47 s.[18]

TYPES OF FOAM

Foams can have different properties depending on the mode of preparation and the gas to air ratio (dilution factor). A higher concentration of sclerosant produces more viscous foam, which is more powerful and suitable for use in larger-caliber veins. Viscous foams or dry foams tend to break on passage through a needle. Liquid foam or wet foam which is created by using a lower concentration of sclerosant should be used for smaller vessels to reduce adverse events.[19]

REQUIREMENTS

- 1-mL and 3-mL syringes for sclerosant
- Three-way stopcock to create foam (Fig. 8.2)
- 25 G, 27 G, 30 G and 32 G disposable needles (27 G needle allows for quicker instillation of larger foam volumes)
- Detergent sclerosant

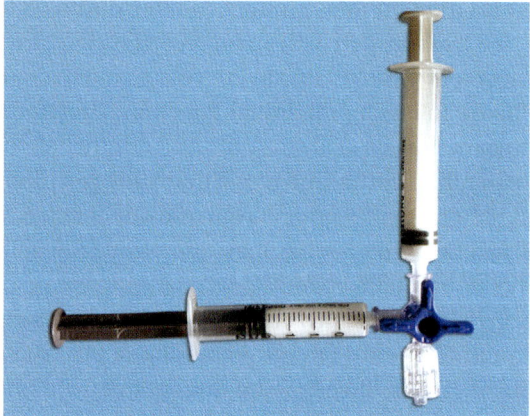

Fig. 8.2: Foam preparation.

- Compression-foam pads, cotton balls, dental roll
- Compression stockings—Class I (20–30 mm Hg) for spider and reticular veins, Class II (30–40 mm Hg) for varicose veins
- In the exceptional case that a severe allergic reaction occurs following treatment, suitable drugs and equipment must be available to manage this problem
- Adjustable table

PATIENT POSITION

Placing the patient in Trendelenburg position has certain advantages. Vein emptying is enhanced in this position, which decreases sclerosant dilution by blood. In Trendelenburg position, the air composition of foam will potentially result in caudal distribution of the sclerosant; thus delaying emptying, increased vein wall contact time and also impedes fast penetration into deep venous system.[20,21]

SCLEROSING AGENTS

Foaming is unique to detergent sclerosants like polidocanol and sodium tetradecyl sulfate.

INDICATIONS AND CONTRAINDICATIONS

Indications and contraindications for foam sclerotherapy do not differ from sclerotherapy with fluid sclerosants. In the case of large varicose veins and recurrent varicose veins, the result obtained with foam sclerotherapy is better than those with fluid sclerotherapy. Favorable results were also reported for venous malformations.[22] Foam can be used for spider veins, but there can be excessive inflammation with treatment of vessels of this size. Fluid foam is preferred for spider veins compared to viscous foam.[20]

The only absolute contraindications are hypersensitivity to sclerosants and obliterated deep veins.

PROCEDURE

The basic rule for injection sclerotherapy is to treat larger veins first before cutaneous veins. Injection with liquid sclerosant should proceed from proximal leg veins and progress distally. The reverse pattern, distal to proximal, is recommended with foam therapy. This change in sclerotherapy technique is because of vasospasm created with foam. The more distal veins subsequently will not be visualized if one starts proximally, and hence, require treatment at a later date when visible.[20]

Punctures should always be made at the safest and most easily accessible site. The puncture site in the case of valvular insufficiency in the saphenous veins should have a distance of at least 10 cm away from the saphenous junction. When sclerosing large veins, irrespective of the concentration, a total amount of foam of 6–8 mL/session or 1–2 mL per injection should not be exceeded.[15] No more than 3 mL is required for the lesser saphenous vein (Tessari).[21] Phlebologists recommend no more than 0.5 mL of foam per injection into telangiectasias and reticular veins. The necessary volume of foam can be estimated from the diameter and length of vein.[7]

The problem with large diameter veins is that foam floats and moves to upper part of vein. This can be reduced by reducing the size of the vein by compression, leg elevation, induction of vasospasm, injection of 10–30 mL normal saline perivenously.[23]

Preferably ultrasound guidance should be used with injection of larger varicosities. Ultrasound-guided foam sclerotherapy is an effective treatment adjunct for nonvisible subcutaneous varicosities and perforator veins. The acoustic shadowing of the foam injected will be readily appreciated on ultrasound imaging. The foam air/sclerosant mix can be tracked to determine which veins have not had exposure and require additional foam to be injected.[15]

Uses of long catheters with balloon tips are more prevalent due to increased efficacy; however, there may be an increased incidence of deep vein thrombosis due to passage through perforators even though foam is reaspirated.[24]

The recommendations now are to inject the GSV at proximal thigh if using direct puncture technique and distal to knee if using long catheters.[7]

Vasospasm is created by the foam used in the reticular veins and therefore compression is not needed during the treatment session. Direct compression after injection is reserved for larger varicose veins.

Table 8.1: Volume in cm³ of a venous segment calculated from the formula of cylinder.

Vein Diameter (cm)	Vein Length (cm)							
	5	7	10	15	20	25	30	35
1.00	3.93	5.50	7.85	11.78	15.71	19.63	23.56	27.49
0.90	3.18	4.45	6.36	9.54	12.72	15.90	19.09	22.27
0.80	2.51	3.52	5.03	7.54	10.05	12.57	15.08	17.59
0.70	1.92	2.69	3.85	5.77	7.70	9.62	11.55	13.47
0.60	1.41	1.98	2.83	4.24	5.65	7.07	8.48	9.90
0.50	0.98	1.37	1.96	2.95	3.93	4.91	5.89	6.87
0.40	0.63	0.88	1.26	1.88	2.51	3.14	3.77	4.40
0.30	0.35	0.49	0.71	1.06	1.41	1.77	2.12	2.47
0.20	0.16	0.22	0.31	0.47	0.63	0.79	0.94	1.10

Source: Goldman MP, Guex J-J, Wu D. Clinical methods for sclerotherapy of varicose veins. In: Goldman M, Weiss R (Eds). Sclerotherapy: Treatment of Varicose and Telangiectatic Leg Veins (5th edition). Saunders Elsevier; 2011. pp. 242-7.

POSTPROCEDURE

Once the session is completed, the leg is compressed with an elastic crepe bandage from ankle to thigh, worn until the following morning. Before applying compression therapy, some minutes should be allowed to avoid premature displacement of the sclerosing foam into other regions. This is followed by thigh-high class I compression stockings worn during the day for a minimum of 3 days and preferably up to 3 weeks during the day. The biggest impact stocking use has is on decreasing hyperpigmentation and vessel clearing. Patients are advised to walk daily to help decrease superficial vein hypertension. Treadmill or elliptical use is allowed. Patients are instructed to avoid all high-impact activities and weight lifting for 1 week.[25]

Vessel Wall Events Following Sclerotherapy[7]

After injection of the foam sclerosant, blood is displaced by the bubbles resulting in contact of the sclerosant with the endothelium. Clinically this is apparent as vasospasm within seconds or minutes, erythema of feeding telangiectasia or no immediate visible changes.

After several days, venous inflammation results in thickening of vessel wall, evident clinically by induration, erythema and tenderness.

Months later fibrosis results resulting in decrease in the diameter of vein and disappearance of varicosity. At times, complete clearance of the varicose veins does not take place, owing to either partial or total recanalization of the treated vein.

Foam Evolution Following Injection

After injection into an isolated segment, a plug of foam is created which remains in contact with endothelium and causes vasospasm. As it is forced from the contracting vein segment, it mixes with blood, gets diluted, bubbles scatter and sclerosant is deactivated by attachment to plasma proteins. So when bubbles are found in remote sites like the lung, heart or brain, they only consist of air and do not carry detectable amounts of sclerosing agent or have any sclerosing properties.[26]

COMPLICATIONS

The adverse effects of foam sclerotherapy are comparable with sclerotherapy using fluid sclerosants. After injection of foam, the foamed sclerosant remains locally in the venous segment to be sclerosed for a longer period of time and provokes a stronger sclerosing effect, which might cause more inflammation, hyperpigmentation and skin necrosis.

- Transient visual disturbances, especially in migraine patients, seem to be a bit more frequent with foam sclerotherapy.[20]
- The active foam can be moved in the vein toward the deep venous system or other venous regions. Improper use therefore might lead to a higher amount of deep venous thrombosis and to sclerosing activity in regions which are not thought to be treated.[20] Hill et al. showed that leg elevation, but not manual pressure of the SFJ, decreased the migration of foam in sclerotherapy.[10] An overall 71.79% decrease in bubble-related side effects (as compared to room air) was attributed to the carbon dioxide foam.[27]
- A rare complication of foam sclerotherapy is the appearance of neurologic symptoms if there is a patent foramen ovale. Foam injected in the leg veins rapidly finds its way to the right side of the heart and may be a factor in producing visual disturbances. The problem may lie with the nitrogen in air which is relatively insoluble, and replacing this with carbon dioxide can limit the reported side effects of treatment.[27]

According to the French multicenter registry, of 12,173 sessions, the rate of serious complication per session with liquid sclerosant is 0.22% and with foam sclerosant is 0.58%.[28]

ADVANTAGES OF FOAM SCLEROTHERAPY

When using foam sclerotherapy, there is a longer dwell time resulting in extended contact period with the vessel wall.[29] The foam displaces blood from the vein creating an air block. This prevents rapid dilution and mixing with blood. Lower concentrations of sclerosants can be used to achieve the same results in light of these attributes. Foam sclerotherapy allows for instillation of larger volumes at one site and a longer injection interval, which can be 8 cm or longer thus resulting in fewer injections per session.[20] With liquid sclerosant, it is recommended not to exceed 0.5-1.0 mL at any one injection point and to advance 3-4 cm.

It is reported by the American Society of Dermatologic Surgery in their technology report, 'The advantage of a foam is that the sclerosing power of the solution is increased 2-fold to 3-fold, while decreasing the toxicity 4-fold.' In addition, the use of lower detergent concentrations minimizes the complication risks with extravasation.[30]

In a study by Hamsel et al., follow-up after 3 weeks showed 84% elimination of reflux in the great saphenous vein with foam versus 40% with liquid sclerosant. At 6 months, six recanalizations were found in the liquid group versus two in the foam group. After 1 year, no additional recanalization was observed with either foam or liquid. Side effects did not differ between groups. The investigators concluded that the efficacy of sclerosing foam is a superior therapy when compared with sclerosing liquid.[2]

CONCLUSION

Foam sclerotherapy seems to be a safer alternative to liquid sclerotherapy with lesser number of injections and better efficacy. Foam sclerotherapy is likely to replace all other techniques for sclerotherapy of veins greater than 2 mm in diameter.

REFERENCES

1. Wright D, Gobin JP, Bradbury AW, et al. The Varisolve European Phase III Investigators Group. Varisolve polidocanol microfoam compared with surgery or sclerotherapy in the management of varicose veins in the presence of trunk vein incompetence: European randomized controlled trial. Phlebology. 2006; 21:180e190.
2. Hamel-Desnos C, Desnos P, Wollmann JC, et al. Evaluation of the efficacy of polidocanol in the form of foam compared with liquid foam in sclerotherapy of the great saphenous vein: initial results. Dermatol Surg. 2003;29(12):1170-5.
3. Creton D, Uhl JF. Foam sclerotherapy combined with surgical treatment for recurrent varicose veins: short term results. Eur J Vasc Endovasc Surg. 2007;33(5): 619-24.
4. Foote RR. Varicose Veins. London: Butterworth & Co; 1949. pp. 1-225.

5. Orbach EJ. The thrombogenic activity of foam of a synthetic anionic detergent (sodium tetradecyl sulfate NNR). Angiology. 1950;1:237-43.
6. Cabrera Garido JR, Cabrera Garcia Olmedo JR, Garcia Olmedo Dominguez MA. Nuevo método de esclerosis en las varices tronculares. Patologia Vasculares. 1993;1:55-72.
7. Goldman MP, Guex J-J, Wu D. Clinical methods for sclerotherapy of varicose veins. In: Goldman M, Weiss R (Eds). Sclerotherapy: Treatment of Varicose and Telangiectatic Leg Veins (5th edition). Edinburgh: Saunders Elsevier; 2011. pp. 242-7.
8. Tessari L, Cavezzi A, Frullini A. Preliminary experience with a new sclerosing foam in the treatment of varicose veins. Dermatol Surg. 2001;27:58-60.
9. Monfreux A. Traitement sclérosant des troncs saphéniens et leurs collatérales de gros calibre par la méthode mus. Phlébologie. 1997;50:351-3.
10. Hill D, Hamilton R, Fung T. Assessment of techniques to reduce sclerosant foam migration during ultrasound-guided sclerotherapy of the great saphenous vein. J Vasc Surg. 2008;48:934-9.
11. Trigilia TCS. Foam preparation for sclerotherapy by means of heat application. Int Angiol. 2005;24(S1-3):70.
12. Hu WS. Oxygen transfer in cell culture bioreactors. Cellular Bioprocess Technology. 2004;1-14.
13. Frullini A, Cavezzi A. Sclerosing foam in the treatment of varicose veins and telangiectases: history and analysis of safety and complications. Dermatol Surg. 2002;28:11.
14. Redondo P, Cabrera J. Microfoam treatment of Klippel-Trénaunay syndrome and vascular malformations. J Am Acad Dermatol. 2008;59:355-6.
15. Smith CP. Foam and liquid sclerotherapy for varicose veins. Phlebology. 2009; 24(Suppl 1):62-72.
16. Rao J, Goldman MP. Stability of foam in sclerotherapy: differences between sodium tetradecyl sulfate and polidocanol and the type of connector used in the double-syringe system technique. Dermatol Surg. 2005;31:19-22.
17. Lai SW, Goldman MP. Does the relative silicone content of different syringes affect the stability of foam in sclerotherapy? J Drugs Dermatol. 2008;7:399-400.
18. Shirazi AR, Goldman M. The use of a 5-mm filter hub increases foam stability when using the double syringe technique. Dermatol Surg. 2008;34:91-2.
19. Breu FX, Guggenbichler S. European consensus meeting on foam sclerotherapy, April 4–6 2003, Tegernsee Germany. Dermatol Surg. 2004;30:709-17.
20. Dietzek CL. Sclerotherapy: introduction to solutions and techniques. Perspect Vasc Surg Endovasc Ther. 2007;19:317-24.
21. Rabe E, Pannier-Fischer NF, Gerlach NH, et al. Guidelines for sclerotherapy of varicose veins. Dermatol Surg. 2004;30:687-93.
22. Yamaki T, Nozaki M, Fujiwara O, et al. Duplex-guided foam sclerotherapy for the treatment of the symptomatic venous malformations of the face. Dermatol Surg. 2002;28:619-22.
23. Thibault P. Internal compression (peri-venous compression) following ultrasound guided sclerotherapy to the great and small saphenous veins. Aust N Z J Phlebol. 2005;9:29.
24. Cavezzi A, Tessari L. Foam sclerotherapy techniques: different gases and methods of preparation, catheter versus direct injection. Phlebology. 2009;24:247.
25. Goldman MP. How to utilize compression after sclerotherapy. Dermatol Surg. 2002;28:860-2.

26. Rush JE, Wright DD. More on microembolism and foam sclerotherapy. N Engl J Med. 2008;359:656.
27. Morrison N, Neuhardt DL, Rogers CR, et al. Comparisons of side effects using air and carbon dioxide foam for endovenous chemical ablation. J Vasc Surg. 2008;47:830-6.
28. Guex JJ. Complications of sclerotherapy: an update. Dermatol Surg. 2010;36 (Suppl 2):1056-63.
29. Jia X, Mowatt G, Burr JM, et al. Systematic review of foam sclerotherapy for varicose veins. Br J Surg. 2007;94:925-36.
30. American Society for Dermatologic Surgery. Available from: http://www.asds-net.org/Media/PositionStatements/technology-Foam_Sclero.html.

CHAPTER 9

Complications of Sclerotherapy

Teresita S Ferrariz, Agnes E Thaebtharm

INTRODUCTION

Successful sclerotherapy results to the sclerosis of the injected vessel.[1] Over the past several years, alarming reports about the complications or adverse events of sclerotherapy have been published. Various mechanisms have been hypothesized.[2] To date, documented severe complications like neurologic and thrombotic events are rare in occurrence in spite of millions of treated cases.[1-5]

The safety of the method has been proven, with 0.22% and 0.57% of complications occurring after liquid and foam sclerotherapy respectively.[3] Adverse events or complications are preventable and can be minimized by considering factors such as pharmacologic properties of the sclerosant, technique, venous anatomy, physiology and pathology, as well as individual comorbidities.[1-6]

PREVENTION OF COMPLICATIONS

A careful approach to sclerotherapy is essential. A comprehensive understanding of the venous anatomy, physiology and pathology, and the method is key to minimizing the risk for complications.[2,3] A complete diagnostic evaluation, which includes history and physical examination, and duplex ultrasound are required. There should be proper patient selection with full and valid informed consent obtained prior to initiation of treatment. It is also important to consider the indications and contraindications of sclerotherapy (Table 9.1), and the current summary of product characteristics or the prescribing information of the sclerosant.[1-3,7]

The use of ultrasonography allows the adequate visualization of the vasculature and is most useful for recurrent and previously treated veins, as well as venous malformations. Ultrasound-guided sclerotherapy (UGS) has been used to improve outcome and safety.[1,4,7]

The volume of the sclerosant and technique affect the outcome.[1-6] The maximum dose for each sclerosant should not be exceeded (e.g., 2 mg/kg/day for polidocanol (POL), and 4 mL of 3% solution or 10 mL of other concentrations per session for sodium tetradecyl sulfate (STS)).[1] A higher volume of sclerosant

Table 9.1: Indications and contraindications of sclerotherapy.[4]

Indications	Contraindications
• Incompetent saphenous veins (Grade 1A) • Tributary varicose veins (Grade 1B) • Incompetent perforating veins (Grade 1B) • Reticular varicose veins (Grade 1A) • Telangiectasias (spider veins) (Grade 1A) • Residual and recurrent varicose veins after previous interventions (Grade 1B) • Varicose veins of pelvic origin (Grade 1B) • Varicose veins (refluxing veins) in proximity of leg ulcers (Grade 1B) • Venous malformations (Grade 1B)	***Absolute*** • Known allergy to the sclerosant • Acute deep vein thrombosis and/or pulmonary embolism • Local infection in the area of sclerotherapy or severe generalized infection • Long-lasting immobility and confinement to bed • Known symptomatic right-to-left shunt (e.g., symptomatic patent foramen ovale) ***Relative*** *(individual benefit-risk assessment mandatory)* • Pregnancy • Breast feeding (interrupt breast feeding for 2–3 days) • Severe peripheral arterial occlusive disease • Poor general health • High thromboembolic risk (e.g., history of thromboembolic events, known severe thrombophilia, hypercoagulable state and active cancer) • Acute superficial venous thrombosis • Neurological disturbances, including migraine, following previous foam sclerotherapy

foams should be avoided and each session limited to less than 10 mL to avoid complications. The choice of gas in foam sclerotherapy improves outcome, with less adverse events using low-nitrogen based sclerosants, or CO_2 and CO_2 + O_2.[1-4] Newer methods of injection such as foam washout sclerotherapy[8] have been developed to reduce the complications of foam sclerotherapy.

A cautious technique (foam versus liquid sclerotherapy; low-volume, low-pressure injections; use of compression, post-operative care, etc.), in addition to regular follow-up with appropriate monitoring also reduce complications or adverse events.[1-5,7-10]

COMPLICATIONS

Allergic Reactions (Urticaria, Anaphylaxis and Allergic Contact Dermatitis)

Hypersensitivity reactions can develop with the use of sclerosants such as STS and POL, except for hypertonic saline.[3,4] Urticaria (Fig. 9.1) and local reactions are more common than true anaphylactic reactions, with frequencies ranging from <0.01–0.6% versus <0.01%.[1,4] Urticaria may result from the

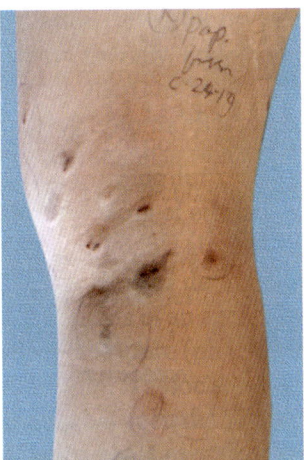

Fig. 9.1: Post-injection urticaria with polidocanol.
Courtesy: Dr Teresita Ferrariz, Makati City, Philippines.

release of perivascular mast cell histamine granules. A generalized urticaria may serve as a clue to an impending anaphylactic reaction.[10] Allergic reactions can be due to either the active agent of the sclerosant or one of its components. Sclerosants using foam have a lower incidence of hypersensitivity reactions compared with liquid, probably due to a lower total volume of allergen exposure.[4] Detergent sclerosing solutions can cause transient bronchospasm with wheezing, and usually resolves spontaneously.[10] The risk factors for anaphylaxis are: multiple previous treatments with liquid sclerosants, history of post-sclerotherapy urticaria and history of asthma exacerbation.[3,4] The most likely sclerosants to cause anaphylaxis are detergents (e.g., morrhuate sodium and ethanolamine oleate), and POL rarely induce systemic urticaria and anaphylaxis.[10] There were four fatal cases of anaphylactic shock reported following the use of STS, and several non-lethal cases were reported with POL. In addition, there was one case of myocardial toxicity reported and one suspected case.[3] A true allergic reaction to adhesives is rare.[4]

Skin Irritation and Bruising

Skin irritation and bruising are expected transient side effects after sclerotherapy.[1,3,4] Irritation leading to blister formation (Fig. 9.2) may be secondary to the compression stockings or bandages, and direct application of compression pads or tapes onto the skin.[1,4,10] The use of these materials on top of an extremely dry skin may lead to irritant contact dermatitis.[4]

Edema and Lymphedema (Superficial Thrombophlebitis)

The incidence of edema is rare (0.5%). It is a transient event resulting from the damage to the superficial saphenous vein (SSV) due to its close proximity with the superficial lymphatic vessels, or secondary to a deep vein occlusion

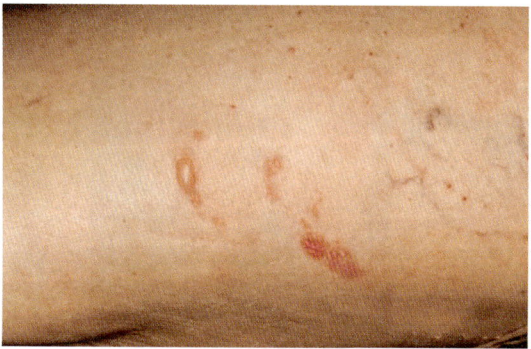

Fig. 9.2: Linear bullae from tape.
Courtesy: Dr Robert Weiss, Baltimore, Maryland, USA.

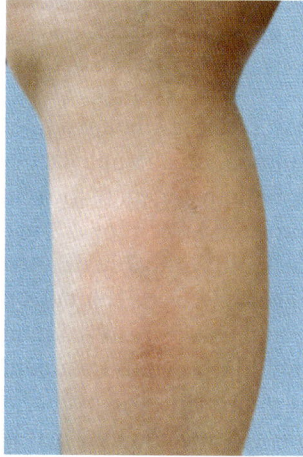

Fig. 9.3: Thrombophlebitis following polidocanol 2% injection.
Courtesy: Dr Teresita Ferrariz, Makati City, Philippines.

from thrombosis or sclerosis. Other risk factors include: extensive sclerotherapy of the superficial incompetent veins followed by occlusion of small segments of lower limb deep veins, obesity, lack of exercise, drugs such as calcium channel blockers and noncompliance to compression therapy.[4] Superficial thrombophlebitis (Fig. 9.3) is characterized by the presence of heat, erythema and tenderness.[10]

Chemical phlebitis post-sclerotherapy can result to a localized lymph stasis presenting as lymphedema. Patients with latent congenital lymphatic system abnormalities are predisposed to having transient lymph stasis following extensive sclerotherapy.[4]

Matting

Telangiectatic matting (Fig. 9.4) occurs in 15–25% of cases and is predominantly seen in women.[4,10] The most common site is the inner distal thigh.[10]

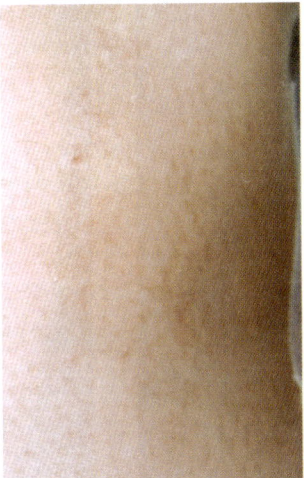

Fig. 9.4: Matting or neovascularization.
Courtesy: Dr Teresita Ferrariz, Makati City, Philippines.

The method (i.e., foam versus liquid sclerotherapy) had no significant effect in matting, although one study reported a slightly higher incidence with POL foam versus POL liquid. This event results from small vessel (<0.2 mm in diameter) proliferation or neovascularization after treatment. The proposed mechanism for this is an excessive sclerotherapy reaction, which can either be due to large volume, high concentration, excessive pressure of injection, or excessive vein obstruction with subsequent angiogenesis.[1,3,4,10] Matting can also be due to inadequate or no treatment of an underlying reflux.[1,4] Additional risk factors include: hormonal supplementation or hormone replacement therapy, obesity, family history of telangiectasias and spider veins, and treatment techniques that result in inflammation.[4,10] Matting can resolve spontaneously in about 3–12 months, but may be permanent.[10]

Pigmentation

Post-sclerotherapy pigmentation (Figs. 9.5A and B) is the persistent pigmentation along the course of the treated blood vessel.[10] Pigmentation results from hemosiderin accumulation and deposition after excessive superficial clotting, inadequate thrombectomy, or melanogenesis secondary to an inflammatory condition.[3,4,10] The incidence for pigmentation ranges from 0.3 to 30%, with higher frequencies occurring with foam.[1] There was no difference in the severity of hyperpigmentation with STS versus POL.[4] There is a higher incidence using stronger sclerosants and at a higher concentration of these agents.[10] Risk factors for post-sclerotherapy pigmentation include: general health of the patient, skin type, size and depth of treated vessels, location of the vessel (below the thighs), medications (e.g., minocycline),

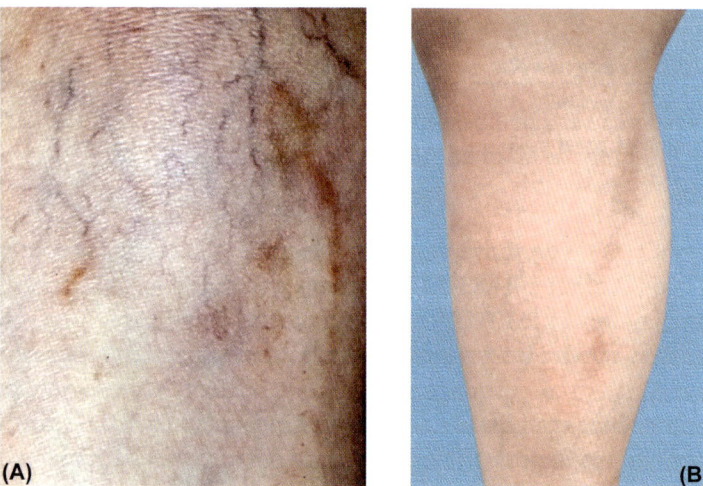

Figs. 9.5A and B: (A) Post-sclerotherapy hyperpigmentation and (B) Post-sclerotherapy hyperpigmentation. *Courtesy:* (A) Dr Agnes Thaebtharm, Manila, Philippines and (B) Dr Teresita Ferrariz, Makati City, Philippines.

presence of a long-standing reflux or stasis dermatitis, vessel fragility, sensitivity to histamines, type and concentration of sclerosant, inadequate or poor treatment technique, inadequate post-treatment compression, high ferritin levels or defects in iron transport and presence of a retained coagulum.[4,10] This complication spontaneously resolves within weeks to months, 90% of cases resolving within 1 year and 10% becoming permanent hyperpigmentation.[1,3,11] Patients with skin types IV, V, and VI should be informed about the possibility of permanent hyperpigmentation and should defer treatment at least 6 months from the last treatment session.[10]

Neurologic Complications (Stroke, Transient Ischemic Attack, Migraine, Visual Disturbances and Nerve Injury)

Neurologic adverse events after sclerotherapy are considered rare (0–2%). Foam sclerotherapy has been more commonly associated with stroke or cerebrovascular accidents (CVA), transient ischemic attacks (TIA), migraines, and visual disturbances (median rate 1.4%), compared to liquid sclerotherapy.[1-5,10,12]

Cerebrovascular accidents and TIA are considered severe complications occurring within minutes to hours, up to days (maximum 5 days).[2-5] Patients who had foam sclerotherapy with subsequent immediate onset strokes were due to a paradoxical gas embolism, while those with delayed onset strokes were due to a paradoxical clot embolism.[1,3,4,13] Risk factors that lead to these complications are the following: foam sclerotherapy, high-volume injection of sclerosants and a patent foramen ovale (PFO) or right-to-left shunt (RLS).[3-5] The choice between the Monfreux method, which creates larger bubbles and the Tessari technique, which produces compact and smaller air bubbles, also affect outcome. The creation of larger bubbles results to a higher likelihood of CVA or TIA.[2,3,5] A higher volume of foam also leads to distant thrombotic and ischemic complications, hence should be avoided.[1,4] The majority of reported cases of stroke or TIA were consistent with findings of a PFO.[2-5,10,12,13] The hypothesized pathophysiology of TIA or CVA after sclerotherapy are: (1) the presence of foam particles reaching the cerebral circulation through a RLS, demonstrated using transcranial Doppler and showed foam bubbles in the middle cerebral artery (although 42% demonstrating bubbles had no sequelae); and (2) an inflammatory reaction to the sclerosing agent, leading to vasospasm.[5]

Visual disturbances and transient migraine-like symptoms are considered the most common adverse events.[1-3] Visual disturbances, such as blurred vision, gray veil, and scotoma, are similar to migraine with aura. A RLS has also been associated with such complications.[2-5,10] The proposed pathophysiology for these include: (1) the presence of microemboli of bubbles to the left circulation through a PFO or another RLS, and (2) the presence of circulating endothelin (endothelin-1) locally released from the injection reaction.[1-4] Endothelin in the cerebral cortex leads to cortical spreading depression, resulting to migraine.[1,2,5] The endothelin level has also been found to be higher among those injected with foam sclerosants.[5] Also, high levels of serotonin (a vasoconstrictor) has been implicated in the pathogenesis of migraine.[4]

Motor and sensory nerve injury occurs in 0.02% of cases.[1,3,4] Injuries presenting as dysesthesia and paresthesia can result from an extravascular injection close to a nerve, especially in the area of the popliteal fossa and calf, where the tibial and sural nerves are intimately associated with the SSV.[3,4,10] The SSV lies very close to the sciatic nerve in the area of the mid-thigh and leakage of sclerosants into this site can cause severe sequelae.[10] Injury to the nerves can be avoided by an in-depth understanding the anatomy of the vessels and with the use of UGS.[3,4]

Thrombotic Events (Deep Vein Thrombosis, Pulmonary Embolism and Superficial Thrombosis)

Thrombotic complications (Figs. 9.6A and B) arise from an inadvertent clot formation at distant portions of the venous system. The incidence of these events ranges from 0.01 to 3.2%, with higher incidence for foam sclerotherapy, and those treated with POL. Most cases of deep vein thrombosis (DVT) occur in distal locations (i.e., lower legs).[1-4,14]

Thrombotic reactions are usually related to a high volume of sclerosing agent, and lowering the dose (≤ 10 mL of foam sclerosant) can reduce the risk specifically for DVT.[3,4,15] The treatment of the small saphenous vein (SSV),

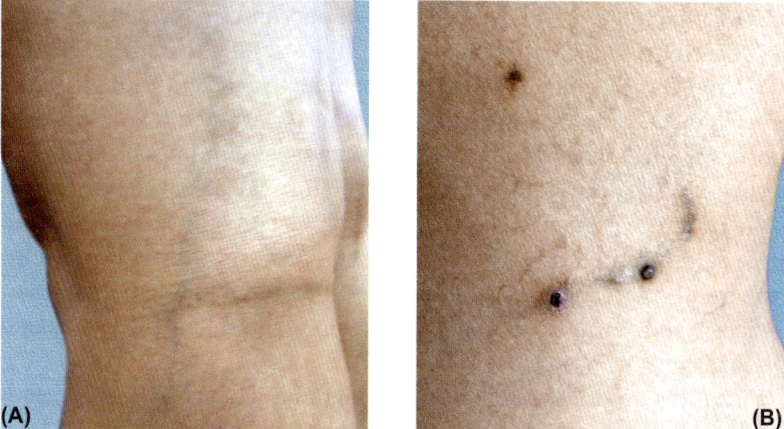

Figs. 9.6A and B: (A) Thrombus formation (blood coagulum) and (B) Thrombus formation. *Courtesy:* Dr Teresita Ferrariz, Makati City, Philippines and (B) Dr Agnes Thaebtharm, Manila, Philippines.

which is highly variable in terms of anatomy, predisposes to DVT. However, the incidence of DVT can be reduced when complete assessment of the deep venous system using ultrasonography was done, and when the type of treated veins are selected carefully.[14,15] Other risk factors for thromboembolic events are: history of thrombophilia or previous thromboembolism, overweight and lack of mobility.[1-3]

Pulmonary embolism (PE) and superficial venous thrombosis (SVT) are very rare, with two cases of PE and three cases of SVT reported.[2,4,16] The postulated pathophysiology of PE is the migration of the sclerosing agent into the pulmonary vasculature resulting to an acute inflammatory reaction or chemical injury to the vessel wall leading to thrombus formation.[16] The diagnosis of SVT is based on the co-presence of an inflammatory component, and that an SVT without inflammation is under diagnosed among sclerotherapy patients.[4]

Necrosis

The incidence for skin necrosis (Figs. 9.7A to D) is very rare, ranging from less than 0.01% to 0.2%.[1,15] Tissue necrosis results from extravasation of the sclerosant into the perivascular area (most common[10]), inadvertent arteriolar injection, vasospasm and excessive compression or traction with tapes.[4,10] Necrosis is most likely with chemical irritants and osmotic agents rather than with detergent sclerosants.[4] Detergent sclerosing agents cause tissue necrosis mainly via arterial occlusion secondary to an inadvertent intra-arterial injection or a veno-arterial reflex vasospasm. A high-speed or high-pressure injection into small vessels can result to a rapid dilation of the target vein and vasospasm of the associated arteries, producing tissue infarction and eventual necrosis.[4,10] The posterior medial malleolar area is the most common site

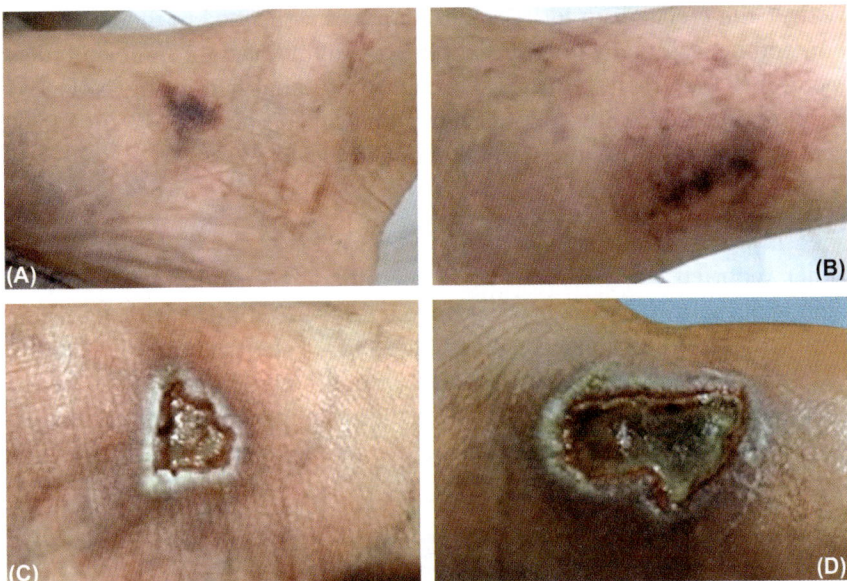

Figs. 9.7A to D: (A and B) Impending skin necrosis with (C and D) subsequent ulceration.
Courtesy: Dr Agnes Thaebtharm, Manila, Philippines.

for inadvertent arterial injection, injuring most commonly the posterior tibial artery. Other common sites are the saphenofemoral and saphenopopliteal junctions. A cutaneous pressure of more than 20 mm Hg decreases the subcutaneous tissue flow in the leg, producing tissue anoxia and localized skin ulcers.[10] Sudden severe pain is the presenting symptom of necrosis secondary to accidental intra-arterial injections. The risk can be minimized with the help of UGS and avoidance of high-volume injections (Grade 1C).[1,4]

Embolia cutis medicamentosa, also known as Nicolau phenomenon is a rare cause of skin necrosis that can be associated with extravenous injection of sclerosants or a backflow to the arterial circulation.[1,3]

Infection

Only a few cases of infection have been reported prior to the use of air foam sclerotherapy; however, there is no evidence of increased incidence with this method. Complications may have resulted from intravenous injection, however, not specific to sclerotherapy.[3]

Recurrence

The recanalization rate over varying periods of follow-up ranges from 10% to 28%, with higher rates (>50%) associated with a longer follow-up period.[17] Recanalization was reported as early as two weeks and with an associated reflux.[15,18] Ulcer recurrence rate was 2.3% after one year, and 5.1% after two years.[18] The mechanism for recanalization was associated to the inflammation and neovascularization present in areas of induced thrombi, and ulcer recurrence was secondary to the reflux and/or recanalization. The risk factors for ulcer recurrence are: superficial hypertension secondary to a superficial venous reflux, lack of exercise and limited leg elevation.[18,19]

Other Complications

Other reported complications after sclerotherapy include transient gross hemoglobinuria (34%) and transient oliguria (57%), arteriovenous fistula (one case report), retained coagulum (7.8–55.1%), chest tightness (<0.004%), vasovagal fainting, compartment syndrome, pulmonary arterial hypertension and metallic taste. Risk factors for these complications are: technique, large volumes of sclerosants, treatment of multiple locations and inadequate visualization of the vasculature.[1-4,17,20]

MANAGEMENT OF COMPLICATIONS

Allergic Reactions

Allergic reactions are not preventable, however, these can be minimized with avoidance of risks.[1,4] The use of latex-free syringes can minimize the incidence of reactions to STS. Urticaria can be managed using potent topical steroids applied immediately after treatment to shorten the time to vessel resolution. Patients with asthma should be treated appropriately with bronchodilators and observed closely for 15 minutes.[10] For anaphylactic reactions, injections should be stopped immediately and followed by the emergency protocol for anaphylaxis [including oxygen and epinephrine (0.2–0.5 mL in 1:1000) when appropriate]. The approach to management is individualized.[1,4,10]

Edema and Lymphedema

A careful technique to avoid phlebitis and deep vein occlusion minimizes the risk to these complications. Compression therapy post-sclerotherapy (up to 1 week), manual lymphatic drainage and bandaging, and lifestyle changes (exercise and weight loss) are recommended. It is also necessary to rule out other causes of edema and lymphedema such as systemic diseases. Lymphatic system scintigraphy can help identify lymphedema.[4]

Matting and Pigmentation

Matting can be prevented by addressing the underlying reflux (with the aid of duplex study), and use of low-concentration sclerosants or phlebectomy to treat any residual patent veins. In addition, the lowest possible volume and the lowest pressure should be used to prevent this complication.[4,10] Patients can be given mild anti-inflammatory creams, and observed at 6 to 8-week intervals until resolution. If matting persists despite the absence of a feeding vessel, the vessels that make up the telangiectatic matting can be treated with sclerotherapy using insulin syringes and 33-gauge needles.[10] Laser and light devices do not treat the underlying reflux, hence are ineffective options.[4]

Pigmentation can be prevented with avoidance of UV exposure (minimum 2 weeks post-procedure), and treatment of intravascular clots using needle aspiration or stab incision (Grade 1C) (Fig. 9.9).[1,4,11] Other treatment options include: exfoliation (e.g., TCA), chelation, topical bleaching agents, 570 nm intense pulsed light (IPL) (4 ms single pulse and 30 J/cm^2), IPL with

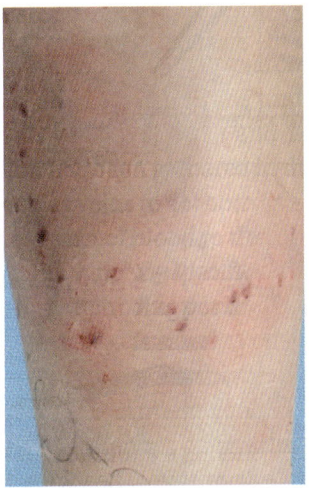

Fig. 9.8: Blood extravasation with surrounding erythema using glycerin 72% + lidocaine-epinephrine (1:2) injection for telangiectasia.
Courtesy: Dr Teresita Ferrariz, Makati City, Philippines.

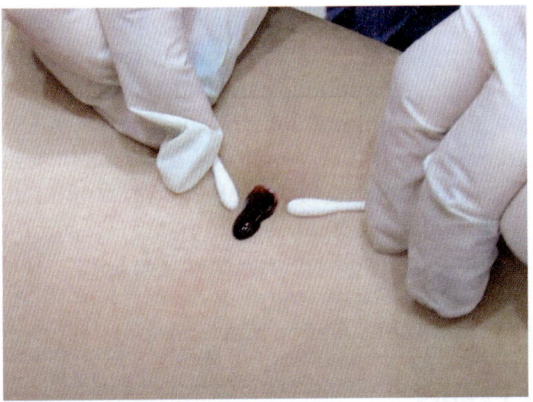

Fig. 9.9: Manual extraction of blood coagulum after stab incision.
Courtesy: Dr Teresita Ferrariz, Makati City, Philippines.

Table 9.2: Approach to minimizing occurrence of telangiectatic matting and post-sclerotherapy hyperpigmentation.[10]	
Telangiectatic matting	**Hyperpigmentation**
• Use minimal sclerosant concentrations • Limit blanching per injection to an area 1–2 cm in diameter • Use low injection pressures to avoid backup of solution into capillaries • Encourage weight loss prior to institution of therapy • Consider discontinuing oral contraceptives or hormonal replacement therapy for the duration of treatment	• Eliminate high-pressure reflux before treating smaller vessels • Minimize risks of vessel rupture • Avoid excessive syringe pressure • Minimize intravascular pressure by elevating leg during treatment • Select a sclerosant with the least inflammatory effects • Use a sclerosant concentration appropriate for vessel size • Apply compression immediately post-treatment • Remove post-sclerotherapy coagulation as early as possible • Avoid concomitant use of minocycline • Direct treatment at the deepest site in a telangiectatic cluster • Avoid treating patients with known defects in iron transport

RF (90.48% efficacy), and other laser therapy (1,064 nm Q-switched laser with nanosecond pulses, 511 nm copper vapor laser, or 510 nm flashlamp-excited pulsed dye laser).[1,4,10,11]

Approach to minimizing post-sclerotherapy telangiectatic matting and hyperpigmentation is summarized in Table 9.2.[10]

Neurologic Complications

Patients who had previous neurological symptoms such as migraine after a previous sclerotherapy should avoid injection of large volumes of foam (<10 mL) or perform liquid sclerotherapy instead (Grade 2C). Patients should remain lying down for a minimum of 5 minutes and avoid Valsalva maneuvers after injection (Grade 2C). A benefit-risk assessment should be done on a case-by-case basis, and referral to neurology and/or ophthalmology service as needed.[1,2,4,5] Active management of neuropathy is recommended with the use of local infiltration of corticosteroids and anesthetics, nonsteroidal anti-inflammatory drugs (NSAIDs), neurotropic drugs, physiotherapy, nerve conduction studies, surgical consultation and long-term follow-up.[4,21]

Thrombotic Events

Early detection and treatment of thrombotic complications like DVT demonstrate constant recovery. Management includes low molecular weight heparin and oral anticoagulation (given for up to 3 months). SVT is treated with NSAIDs and compression therapy, and anticoagulants in select cases. A complete duplex check of the deep and muscular venous system is recommended in case of abnormal symptoms after foam sclerotherapy. High-risk patients with DVT or thrombophilia history should use thromboprophylaxis in line with the current guidelines or recommendations (Grade 1C). Physical prophylaxis such as compression therapy and exercise, in addition to low-volume injections are recommended (Grade 1C). A benefit-risk assessment on a case-by-case basis should also be performed.[1-4]

Necrosis

The onset of sudden and severe pain should herald immediate withdrawal of injection.[1,4,10] Extravasated sclerosants can be diluted with saline, however, this can further increase the incidence of necrosis. Instead, dilution with a hyaluronidase solution (300 USP units hyaluronidase in 5 mL 0.9% sodium chloride) can be attempted.[10] A local catheter-directed anticoagulation and thrombolysis could be started if warranted. Systemic anticoagulation is given in cases of intra-arterial injections.[1,4] Treatment with heparin and fibrinolytic agents (e.g., urokinase, tissue plasminogen activator and glycoprotein IIb-IIIa inhibitors).[10] Further tissue damage can be reduced with early administration of systemic steroid (Grade 1C).[1,4] Other possible treatment options include: IV dextran, cooling of the extremity and local injections of procaine. Compression of more than 30–40 mm Hg at night while the patient is recumbent should be avoided to prevent tissue anoxia and subsequent skin ulceration. Also, traction necrosis is prevented by careful application of the tape and avoidance of excessive traction on the tape. Ulcers can be managed with occlusive or hydrocolloid dressings.[10] VAVR can be treated with topical vasodilating agents such as topical nitrates, oral antiplatelet, systemic anticoagulants and NSAIDs.[1,4] Embolia cutis medicamentosa can be minimized using small-sized syringes.[3]

Recurrence

Retreatment of partially recanalized vein segments is recommended (Grade 1B).[1] Early detection of recanalization is achieved with constant ultrasonographic monitoring.[17]

Infection, Skin Irritation, Injection Site Reactions and Other Complications

Infections are avoided using sterile techniques of injection[3] and treated with appropriate antibiotics. General or local transient reactions, such as skin irritation, chest tightness, vasovagal reactions, metallic taste, retained coagulum and injection site reactions, are avoided by improving general safety. Recommendations include injection of highly viscous foam into varicose veins, avoiding patient or leg movement for a few minutes after injection, and avoiding Valsalva maneuvers (Level 1C).[1] Skin irritation can be treated with topical agents.[4] Contact dermatitis secondary to adhesives can be managed with medium-potency topical steroid applied for one week. A cohesive dressing instead of an adhesive dressing to secure post-treatment compression is advised.[10] Vasovagal reactions are managed by leg elevation (for at least 30 minutes) and injection of 0.25 mg atropine as needed.[3] Transient gross hemoglobinuria and oliguria are treated with generous hydration and alkalinization of urine.[20] AVF management includes observation with regular ultrasonographic monitoring and conservative treatment.[19] Retained coagulum is also prevented by injecting small volumes from single entry points and applying adequate compression.[4]

CONFLICTS OF INTEREST

The authors have no conflicts of interest to declare.

ACKNOWLEDGMENT

Margaret Mary B Alegre, MD; Robert A Weiss, MD, FAAD, FACPh.

REFERENCES

1. Rabe E, Breu FX, Cavezzi A, et al. Guideline Group. European guidelines for sclerotherapy in chronic venous disorders. Phlebology. 2014;29(6):338-54.
2. Guex JJ. Complications and side-effects of foam sclerotherapy. Phlebology. 2009; 24(6):270-4.
3. Guex JJ. Complications of sclerotherapy: an update. Dermatol Surg. 2010;36: 1056-63.
4. Cavezzi A, Parsi K. Complications of foam sclerotherapy. Phlebology. 2012; 27(Suppl 1):46-51.
5. Sarvananthan T, Shepherd AC, Willenberg T, et al. Neurological complications of sclerotherapy for varicose veins. J Vasc Surg. 2012;55:243-51.
6. Albanese G, Kondo K. Pharmacology of sclerotherapy. Semin Intervent Radiol. 2010;27:391-9.
7. Maurya AK, Singh S, Sachdeva V, et al. Outcome of ultrasound guided foam sclerotherapy treatment for varicose veins: procedure is standard and need no further study. Indian J Vasc Endovasc Surg. 2015;2:96-100.
8. Fattahi K. Foam washout sclerotherapy: a new technique geared toward reducing short- and long-term complications of regular foam sclerotherapy and comparison with existing foam sclerotherapy method. J Vasc Surg. 2013;1(1):111.
9. National Institute for Health and Care Excellence. Varicose veins in the legs—the diagnosis and management of varicose veins. (Clinical guideline 168.) 2013. Available from: http://guidance.nice.org.uk/CG168 [Accessed on October 2017].
10. Weiss RA, Weiss MA, Beasley KL. Sclerotherapy and Vein Treatment (2nd edition). New York: McGraw-Hill; 2012. pp. 196-207.

11. Mlosek RK, Wozniak W, Malinowska S, et al. The removal of post-sclerotherapy pigmentation following sclerotherapy alone or in combination with crossectomy. Eu J Vasc Endovasc Surg. 2012;43:100-5.
12. Forlee MV, Grouden M, Moore DJ, et al. Stroke after varicose vein foam injection sclerotherapy. J Vasc Surg. 2006;43:162-4.
13. DeLaney M, Bowe C, Higgins G III. Acute stroke from air embolism after leg sclerotherapy. West J Emerg Med. 2010;11(4)397.
14. Gillet JL, Lausecker M, Sica M, et al. Is the treatment of the small saphenous veins with foam sclerotherapy at risk of deep vein thrombosis? Phlebology. 2014;29(9):600-7.
15. Hemmati H, Toloie M, Esmaeili-Delshad, et al. Complications of sclerotherapy with sclerosing foam in lower extremity varicose veins. Zahedan J Res Med Sci. 2015;17(1):27-9.
16. Oktay V, Yildiz CE, Abaci O, et al. A rare complication of sclerotherapy: pulmonary embolism. Yed Med J. 2012;6(22):506-8.
17. Neto FC, Kessler IM, de Araujo GR. Arteriovenous fistula after ultrasound guided foam sclerotherapy: case report. J Vasc Bras. 2015;14(3):258-61.
18. Howard JK, Slim FJA, Wakely MC, et al. Recanalisation and ulcer recurrence rates following ultrasound-guided foam sclerotherapy. Phlebology. 2015;0(0):1-8.
19. Neto FC, Kessler IM, de Araujo GR. Arteriovenous fistula after ultrasound guided foam sclerotherapy: Case report. J Vasc Bras. 2015;14(3):258-61.
20. Barranco-Pons R, Burrows P, Landrigan-Ossar M, et al. Gross hemoglobinuria and oliguria are common transient complications of sclerotherapy for venous malformations: Review of 475 procedures. AJR. 2012;199(3):691-94.
21. Stuart S, Patel PA, Chippington S, et al. A test of nerves. The incidence of neuropathy following STS sclerotherapy of venous malformations. J Vasc Interven Radiol. 2013;24Suppl(4):77-8.

CHAPTER 10

Sclerotherapy for Cystic and Benign Vascular Lesions

Sacchidanand S, Nagesh TS, Shruthi C

Sclerotherapy is a procedure involving injection of a solution (sclerosant) into a vessel to cause endothelial damage, obliteration of the lumen of the vessel and transform into a fibrous cord that cannot be recanalised.[1]

Sclerotherapy remains the primary treatment for small-vessel varicose disease of the lower extremities. These small vessels include telangiectasias, venulectasias, hemorrhoids, etc.[2] With the knowledge of mechanism of action of sclerosants, the uses of sclerotherapy has been extended to treat cystic conditions like oral mucous retention cysts, vascular lesions like hemangiomas, pyogenic granulomas in the recent past. However, there are only few studies so far to establish the efficacy of sclerotherapy in these conditions.[3-11]

Cystic lesions like sebaceous cysts, oral mucous cysts, lymphangiomas and vascular lesions like pyogenic granulomas, hemangiomas are commonly encountered in dermatological practice. There are various surgical and non-surgical modalities of treatment for the above-mentioned conditions with no clear consensus. Also, surgical methods are associated with significant discomfort, complications and recurrences.

We will briefly discuss the common cystic and vascular lesions encountered in dermatology outpatient departments.

SEBACEOUS CYST/EPIDERMOID CYST

Epidermoid cysts represent the most common cutaneous cysts.

Clinical Presentation

Epidermoid cysts appear as flesh–colored-to-yellowish, firm, round nodules of variable size. A central pore or punctum may be present. Epidermoid cysts are most common (in descending order of frequency) on the face, trunk, neck, extremities and scalp.[12,13]

Sclerotherapy Procedure for Epidermoid Cyst

The authors have tried treating the epidermoid cyst by sclerotherapy. The contents of the cyst are aspirated with a wide bore needle followed by injection

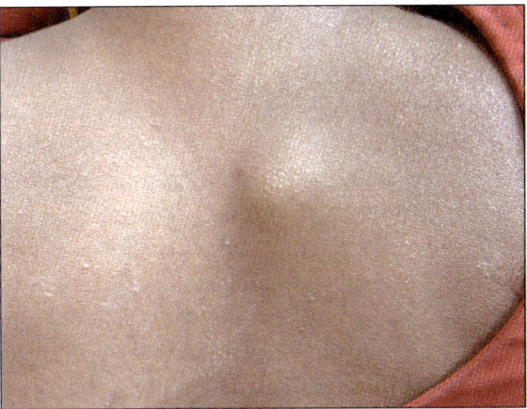

Fig. 10.1: Sebaceous cyst—before treatment.

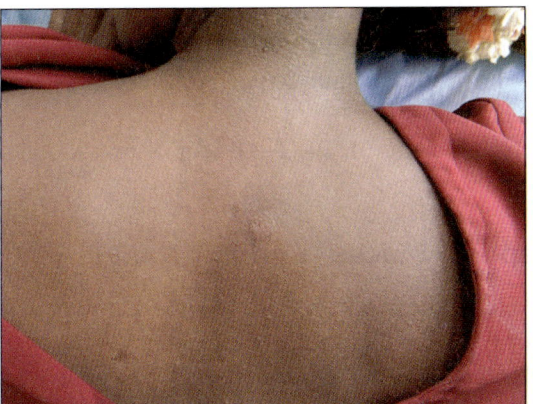

Fig. 10.2: Sebaceous cyst—after treatment.

of sclerosant into the cyst and compression for 3–5 minutes. Sodium tetradecyl sulfate (STS) and polidocanol (POL) were used. Common concentration of the sclerosant used were 1.5% for STS and 3% for POL. Injections can be repeated for two to three times depending on the size of the cyst. An interval of 1 week to 10 days is given between two sittings. Figures 10.1 and 10.2 show the pretreatment and posttreatment results respectively.

MUCOUS CYST AND RANULA

Collectively mucocele, oral ranula and plunging ranula are clinical terms for a pseudocyst that is associated with mucus extravasation into the surrounding soft tissues. These lesions occur as the result of trauma or obstruction to the salivary gland excretory duct and spillage of mucin into the surrounding soft tissues.

Clinical Presentation

Presents as a nontender, mobile, dome-shaped enlargement (0.4–1 cm) with intact epithelium that lies over it. Superficial lesions take on a bluish to translucent hue. The mucosa lining is usually intact; however, repeated sucking on the lesion may result in a white, rough, keratotic surface. Palpation reveals a fluctuant mass that does not blanch on compression.

Although mucocele can occur anywhere in oral cavity, following sites are involved in descending order: lower labial mucosa, floor of mouth, ventral tongue, buccal mucosa, palate and retromolar area.[14]

The oral ranula is a relatively large unilateral blue to translucent mass in the floor of the mouth that remotely resembles the belly of a frog (*Rana* species). The consistency is cystic, and the lesion does not blanch on compression.

Mucoceles and ranulas may spontaneously resolve, especially in infants and young children.[15]

Treatment options include:
- Aspiration, micro-marsupialization technique, laser ablation, cryosurgery and electrocautery[16-20]
- Use of sclerosing agent for the treatment of oral ranulas is considered experimental[21,22]

Sclerotherapy for Mucous Cyst and Ranula

Figures 10.3 to 10.6 show and pre and post treatment results of sclerotherapy for mucous cyst and ranula. The contents of the cyst are evacuated and sclerosant injected into the mucous cyst followed by compression. The patient is asked to follow up after one week and injection may be repeated if needed.

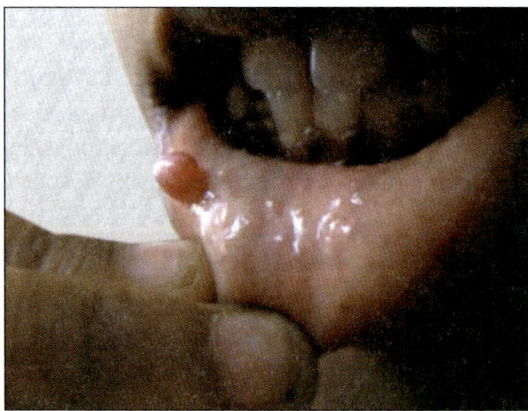

Fig. 10.3: Mucocele—pretreatment.

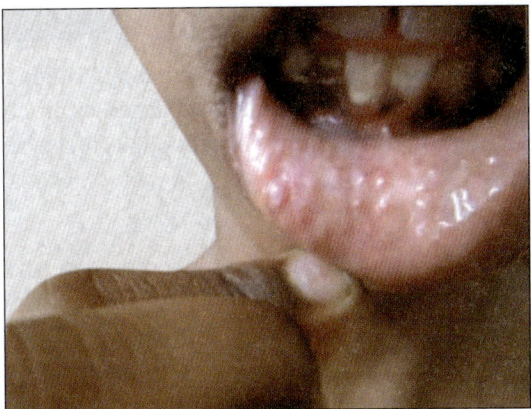

Fig. 10.4: Mucocele—posttreatment.

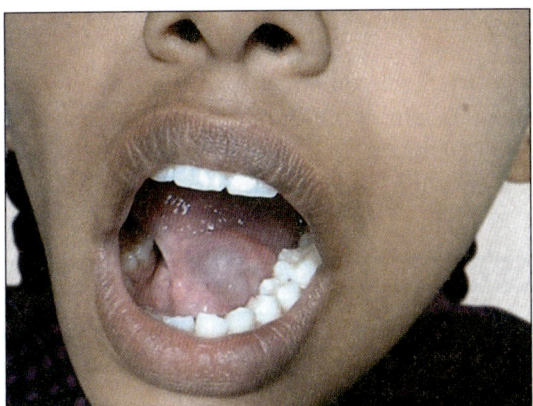

Fig. 10.5: Ranula—before treatment.

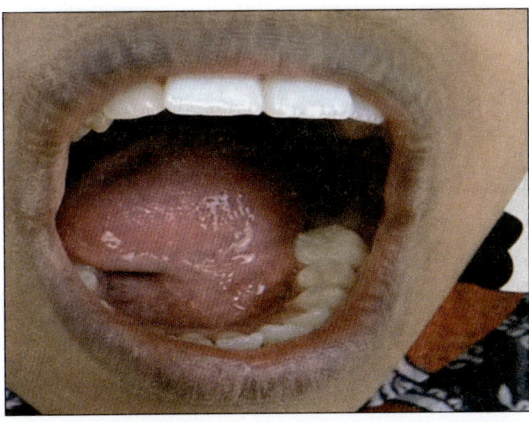

Fig. 10.6: Complete resolution after treatment with 1.5% sodium tetradecyl sulfate (STS).

STEATOCYSTOMA MULTIPLEX

First described by Jamieson[23] in 1873, and coined by Pringle in 1899, steatocystoma multiplex is a disorder of the pilosebaceous unit characterized by the development of numerous sebum-containing dermal cysts.

Clinical Presentation

Lesions present as numerous flesh-to-yellow-colored dermal cysts ranging in size from 3 mm to 3 cm. Individual cysts range from elastic to firm and are freely movable. The lesions lack a central punctum. Cyst contents appear as an odorless creamy or oily fluid. Cysts are distributed in areas where high numbers of sebaceous glands are found—chest, arms, axillae and neck.

Treatment options:
- Cryosurgery, aspiration, excision, carbon dioxide laser.[24-28]

Sclerotherapy

The authors have tried sclerotherapy for the treatment of steatocystoma multiplex with good results. It is a simple procedure with injections of small amounts of either POL or STS in a concentration of 1.5% into the individual cysts after aspiration of the contents of the cyst (Figs. 10.7 and 10.8).

LYMPHANGIOMA CIRCUMSCRIPTUM

Lymphangiomas are rare benign proliferations of the lymphatic system and may be primary (congenital), occurring de novo in early childhood or later in life or secondary (acquired) due to impaired lymphatic flow following destruction of lymphatics due to disease, surgery or radiation. The superficial

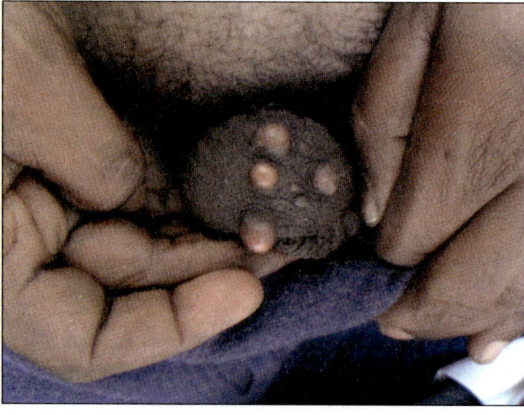

Fig. 10.7: Steatocystoma multiplex.

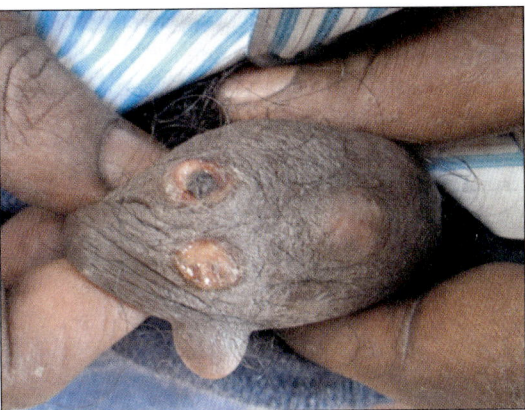

Fig. 10.8: After four sittings of sclerotherapy.

vesicles are called lymphangioma circumscriptum. The more deep seated group includes cavernous lymphangioma and cystic hygroma.[29,30]

Presentation

Usually, lesions are asymptomatic, but, occasionally, patients may have spontaneous episodes of minor bleeding and copious drainage of clear fluid from ruptured vesicles. Lesions are characterized by persistent, multiple clusters of translucent vesicles that usually contain clear lymph fluid (often compared with frog spawn). These vesicles represent superficial saccular dilations from underlying lymphatic vessels that occupy the papilla and push upward against the overlying epidermis. Each skin lesion may range from a minute vesicle to a small bulla-sized lesion. These vesicles can be clear or vary from pink to dark red because of serosanguineous fluid and hemorrhage. These vesicles often are associated with verrucous changes, which give them a warty appearance.[31]

The sites of predilection are the proximal extremities, trunk, axilla and oral cavity, especially the tongue. Involvement in other areas, such as the scrotum, is not uncommon. Lymphangioma circumscriptum has a high recurrence rate after excision because of its deep component.

Investigations

Dermoscopic findings may aid in the diagnosis of cutaneous lymphangioma circumscriptum. Nodules filled with clear fluid show light brown lacunas surrounded by paler septa.[32]

Magnetic resonance imaging (MRI) can help define the degree of involvement and the entire anatomy of the lymphangioma lesion. MRI can help prevent unnecessary extensive, incomplete surgical resection, because of the association with a high recurrence rate.

Treatment

The preferred treatment for lymphangiomas is complete surgical excision. The use of other treatment modalities has been advocated; these include cryotherapy, sclerotherapy, cautery, electrodessication, pulsed-dye laser and vaporization with a carbon dioxide laser.[33]

A new therapeutic option for lymphangioma circumscriptum is sclerotherapy.[33]

Sclerotherapy

Sclerotherapy using STS or POL has shown good results. Usually 1–1.5% of the sclerosing solution can be injected into the lesion (Figs. 10.9 and 10.10).

PYOGENIC GRANULOMA

Pyogenic granuloma (lobular capillary hemangioma) is a relatively common benign vascular lesion of the skin and mucosa. Also known as granuloma gravidarum, eruptive hemangioma, pregnancy tumor, etc. Pyogenic granuloma is a misnomer; they are neither infectious nor granulomatous. Other pyogenic granuloma variants include the disseminated, subcutaneous, intravenous and drug-induced subtypes.[34]

Patients with pyogenic granuloma may report a glistening red lesion that bleeds spontaneously or following irritation. The classic exophytic raspberry-like lesion has a moist surface and an epithelial collarette at the base. Bleeding, erosion, ulceration and crusting frequently are noted. Regressing lesions appear as a soft fibroma.

The head and neck, trunk and distal extremities (especially the fingers) are sites of predilection, but lesions occur anywhere. Oral lesions are most common on the lips, gingiva and tongue.[34] Rare multiple pyogenic granuloma lesions may be grouped or eruptive and disseminated in nature. Congenital disseminated pyogenic granulomas have been reported.[34]

Treatment

- Offending traumatic factor/medication if any to be removed
- Topical timolol or propranolol have both been used to treat pyogenic granulomas

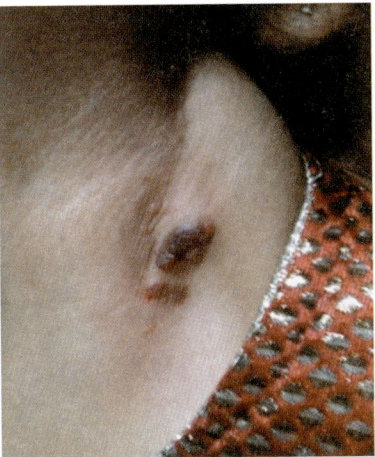

Fig. 10.9: Lymphangioma circumscriptum.

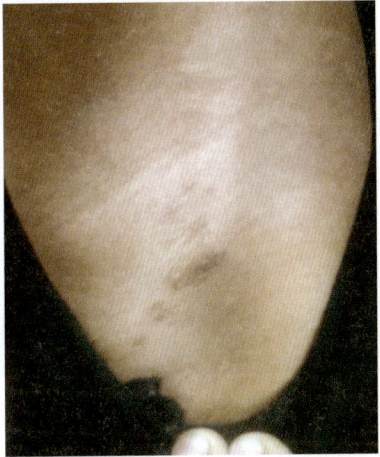

Fig. 10.10: Lymphangioma circumscriptum after five sessions of sclerotherapy.

Surgical Care

Excision, electrocautery, injectable sclerosing agents,[35,36] chemical cauterization with silver nitrate, topical phenol for periungual lesions and photodynamic therapy with 5-aminolevulinic acid intralesional injection have all been used.[34]

Sclerotherapy

Either POL or STS are injected into the lesion till the lesion blanches. Usually 0.1–0.2 mL of the sclerosant is injected depending on the size of the lesion. Pressure might be given around the lesion by placing the ring of the handle

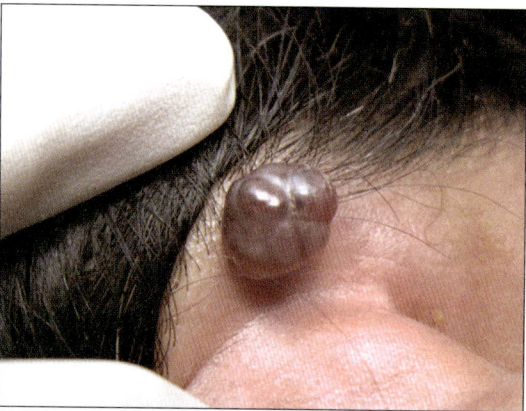

Fig. 10.11: Pyogenic granuloma.

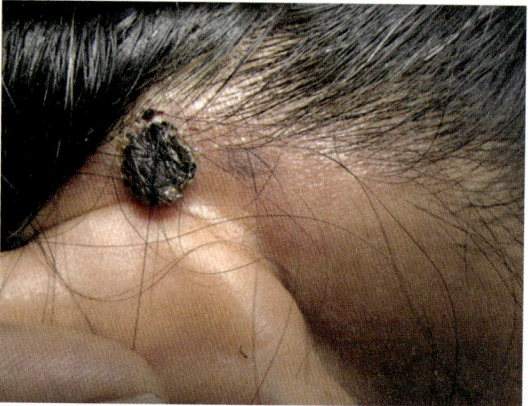

Fig. 10.12: Pyogenic granuloma after one session of sclerotherapy.

of an artery forceps, or by tying thread at the base of the lesion to prevent any inadvertent spread of the sclerosant. Repeated injections might be given after one week. In the authors' experience, most of the lesions respond within one to two sittings (Figs 10.11 and 10.12).

Advantages of Sclerotherapy over Surgical Procedures

- Minimal discomfort to the patient
- Negligible blood loss—procedures like excision and electrocautery can be associated with significant bleeding during the procedure
- Simple procedure
- Minimal surgical expertise is required
- Economical

- Local anesthesia is not needed
- No requirement of postoperative dressings or any specific care
- Better aesthetic results with minimal scarring

ACKNOWLEDGMENTS

We acknowledge Dr Nitin Barde for providing the photographs for Figures 10.1 and 10.2, and Dr Shruti C for providing the clinical photographs for Figures 10.3 to 10.12.

REFERENCES

1. Khunger N, Sacchidanand S. Standard guidelines for care: sclerotherapy in dermatology. Indian J Dermatol Venereol Leprol. 2011;77(2):222-31.
2. Goldman, M. Sclerotherapy treatment of varicose and telangiectatic leg vein (2nd edition). St. Louis: Mosby; 1995.
3. Fukase S, Ohta N, Inamura K, et al. Treatment of ranula wth intracystic injection of the streptococcal preparation OK-432. Ann Otol Rhinol Laryngol. 2003;112(3): 214-20.
4. Carvalho RA, Neto V. Letter: Polidocanol sclerotherapy for the treatment of pyogenic granuloma. Dermatol Surg. 2010;36 (Suppl 2):1068-70.
5. Roh JL, Kim HS. Primary treatment of pediatric plunging ranula with nonsurgical sclerotherapy using OK-432 (Picibanil). Int J Pediatr Otorhinolaryngol. 2008; 72(9):1405-10.
6. Moon SE, Hwang EJ, Cho KH. Treatment of pyogenic granuloma by sodium tetradecyl sulfate sclerotherapy. Arch Dermatol. 2005;141(5):644-6.
7. Chen Z, Zheng J, Zhang S. Intralesional pingyangmycin injection sclerotherapy for oral ranulas. Open J Stomatol. 2013;3:359-64.
8. Sanlialp I, Karnak I, Tanyel FC, et al. Sclerotherapy for lymphangioma in children. Int J Pediatr Otorhinolaryngol. 2003;67(7):795.
9. Khunger N. Combination technique of radiofrequency ablation with sclerotherapy in acquired lymphangiectasis of the vulva. J Cutan Aesthet Surg. 2009;2(1):33-5.
10. Winter H, Drager E, Sterry W. Sclerotherapy for treatment of hemangiomas. Dermatol Surg. 2000;26(2):105-8.
11. Grover C, Khurana A, Sambit N. Bhattacharya sclerotherapy for the treatment of infantile hemangiomas. J Cutan Aesthet Surg. 2012;5(3):201-3.
12. Handa U, Kumar S, Mohan H. Aspiration cytology of epidermoid cyst of terminal phalanx. Diagn Cytopathol. 2002;26(4):266-7.
13. Karacal N, Topal U, Kutlu N. Popliteal epidermoid cyst: an unusual location. Plast Reconstr Surg. 2004;114(3):830-1.
14. Chi AC, Lambert PR 3rd, Richardson MS, et al. Oral mucoceles: a clinicopathologic review of 1,824 cases, including unusual variants. J Oral Maxillofac Surg. 2011;69(4):1086-93.
15. Mínguez-Martinez I, Bonet-Coloma C, Ata-Ali-Mahmud J, et al. Clinical characteristics, treatment, and evolution of 89 mucoceles in children. J Oral Maxillofac Surg. 2010;68(10):2468-71.
16. Zhi K, Wen Y, Ren W, et al. Management of infant ranula. Int J Pediatr Otorhinolaryngol. 2008;72(6):823-6.

17. Delbem AC, Cunha RF, Vieira AE, et al. Treatment of mucus retention phenomena in children by the micro-marsupialization technique: case reports. Pediatr Dent. 2000;22(2):155-8.
18. Jinbu Y, Kusama M, Itoh H, et al. Mucocele of the glands of Blandin-Nuhn: clinical and histopathologic analysis of 26 cases. Oral Surg Oral Med Oral Pathol Oral Radiol Endod. 2003;95(4):467-70.
19. Mintz S, Barak S, Horowitz I. Carbon dioxide laser excision and vaporization of nonplunging ranulas: a comparison of two treatment protocols. J Oral Maxillofac Surg. 1994;52(4):370-2.
20. Neumann RA, Knobler RM. Treatment of oral mucous cysts with an argon laser. Arch Dermatol. 1990;126(6):829-30.
21. Fukase S, Ohta N, Inamura K, et al. Treatment of ranula wth intracystic injection of the streptococcal preparation OK-432. Ann Otol Rhinol Laryngol. 2003; 112(3):214-20.
22. Roh JL, Kim HS. Primary treatment of pediatric plunging ranula with nonsurgical sclerotherapy using OK-432 (Picibanil). Int J Pediatr Otorhinolaryngol. 2008; 72(9):1405-10.
23. Jamieson WA. Case of numerous cutaneous cysts scattered over the body. Edin Med J. 1873;19:223-5.
24. Duzova AN, Senturk GB. Suggestion for the treatment of steatocystoma multiplex located exclusively on the face. Int J Dermatol. 2004;43(1):60-2.
25. Schmook T, Burg G, Hafner J. Surgical pearl: mini-incisions for the extraction of steatocystoma multiplex. J Am Acad Dermatol. 2001;44(6):1041-2.
26. Rossi R, Cappugi P, Battini M, et al. CO_2 laser therapy in a case of steatocystoma multiplex with prominent nodules on the face and neck. Int J Dermatol. 2003; 42(4):302-4.
27. Krahenbuhl A, Eichmann A, Pfaltz M. CO_2 laser therapy for steatocystoma multiplex. Dermatologica. 1991;183(4):294-6.
28. Bakkour W, Madan V. Carbon dioxide laser perforation and extirpation of steatocystoma multiplex. Dermatol Surg. 2014;40(6):658-62.
29. Whimster IW. The pathology of lymphangioma circumscriptum. Br J Dermatol. 1976;94(5):473-86.
30. Patel GA, Siperstein RD, Ragi G, et al. Zosteriform lymphangioma circumscriptum. Acta Dermatovenerol Alp Panonica Adriat. 2009;18(4):179-82.
31. Patel GA, Schwartz RA. Cutaneous lymphangioma circumscriptum: frog spawn on the skin. Int J Dermatol. 2009;48(12):1290-5.
32. Jha AK, Lallas A, Sonthalia S. Dermoscopy of cutaneous lymphangioma circumscriptum. Dermatol Pract Concept. 2017;7(2):37-8.
33. Puri N. Treatment options of lymphangioma circumscriptum. Indian Dermatol Online J. 2015;6(4):293-4.
34. Wollina U, Langner D, França K, et al. Pyogenic Granuloma—a common benign vascular tumor with variable clinical presentation: new findings and treatment options. Open Access Maced J Med Sci. 2017;5(4):423-6.
35. Rahman H. Pyogenic granuloma successfully cured by sclerotherapy: a case report. J Pakistan Association Dermatol. 2016;24(4):361-4.
36. Moon SE, Hwang EJ, Cho KH. Treatment of pyogenic granuloma by sodium tetradecyl sulfate sclerotherapy. Arc Dermatol. 2005;141(5):644-6.

CHAPTER 11

Surgical Treatment of Varicose Veins

Durganna T

INTRODUCTION

The principles of the operation are to ligate the point of junctional incompetence and to remove the refluxing trunk and dilated tributaries. Preoperatively, a careful consent is taken, explaining the risks of infection, minor nerve injury and recurrence, the varicose veins must be tramlined using an indelible marker pen to enable accurate identification varicosities during surgery. The operation is usually performed under general anesthesia but locoregional anesthesia is possible.

HISTORY

The Rindfleisch–Friedel procedure of the early 1900s involved one incision to the level of the deep fascia that wrapped around the leg six times, creating a spiral gutter that brought into view a large number of superficial veins, each one of which was ligated. This wound was left open to heal by granulation.

The Linton procedure, introduced in the late 1930s, used a large linear medial leg incision that brought into view all the superficial and perforator veins of the leg. Incompetent superficial veins were removed, and perforating veins were interrupted.

Friedrich Trendelenburg, in the late 1800s, introduced a mid-thigh ligation of the great saphenous vein (GSV). The outcomes were variable, and the procedure was later modified by his student Perthes, who advocated a groin incision a ligation of the GSV at the saphenofemoral junction (SFJ). Later, even better outcomes were found if stripping of GSV with ligation at the SFJ was performed over ligation alone.

Various methods of stripping are:
- *Extraluminar method* using a vein stripper of the Mayo type
- *Intraluminar method*
    - *By Inversion (Keller method)*—lesser chances of injury to the surrounding soft tissue
    - *By Pleating (concertina method)*—more injury to soft tissue leading to hematoma

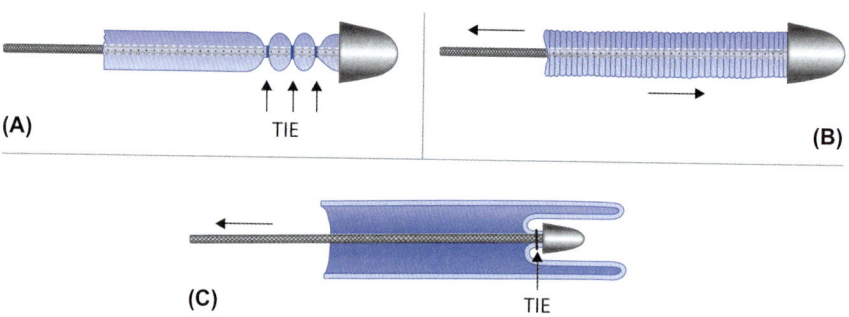

Figs. 11.1A to C: (A) This shows how the vein is secured to the distal end of the stripper. This helps the vein to "concertina" on the wire shaft when traction is made; (B) demonstrates how the vein becomes corrugated against the stripper head at the completion of the operation; (C) shows the method of stripping in which the vein is made to invert during the stripping process. This method has certain disadvantages.

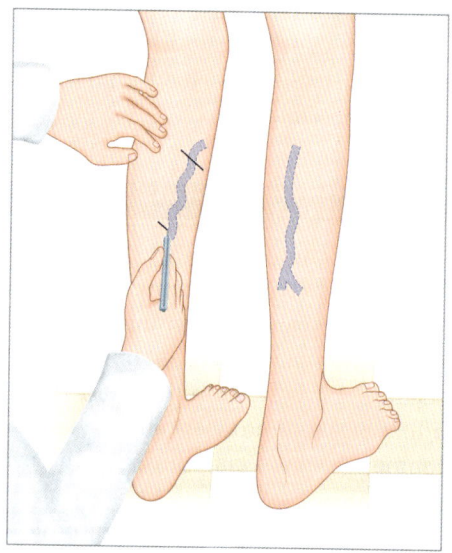

Fig. 11.2: Planning the procedure before surgery. Preoperative marking out of veins by an experienced person is essential to ensure easy identification of veins to be removed. There is no standard procedure—the operation is planned individually for each patient.

SAPHENOFEMORAL LIGATION AND LONG SAPHENOUS STRIPPING (FIGS. 11.3 AND 11.4)

Once the patient is sedated and anesthetized, a small incision is made 2–3 cm distal and lateral to the pubic tubercle. Flush ligation of the SFJ can be done under local anesthesia, but as we nearly always strip the GSV, we rarely perform it. The junction of the GSV with the common femoral vein (i.e., SFJ) is identified and isolated. Anteromedial and posterolateral tributaries are

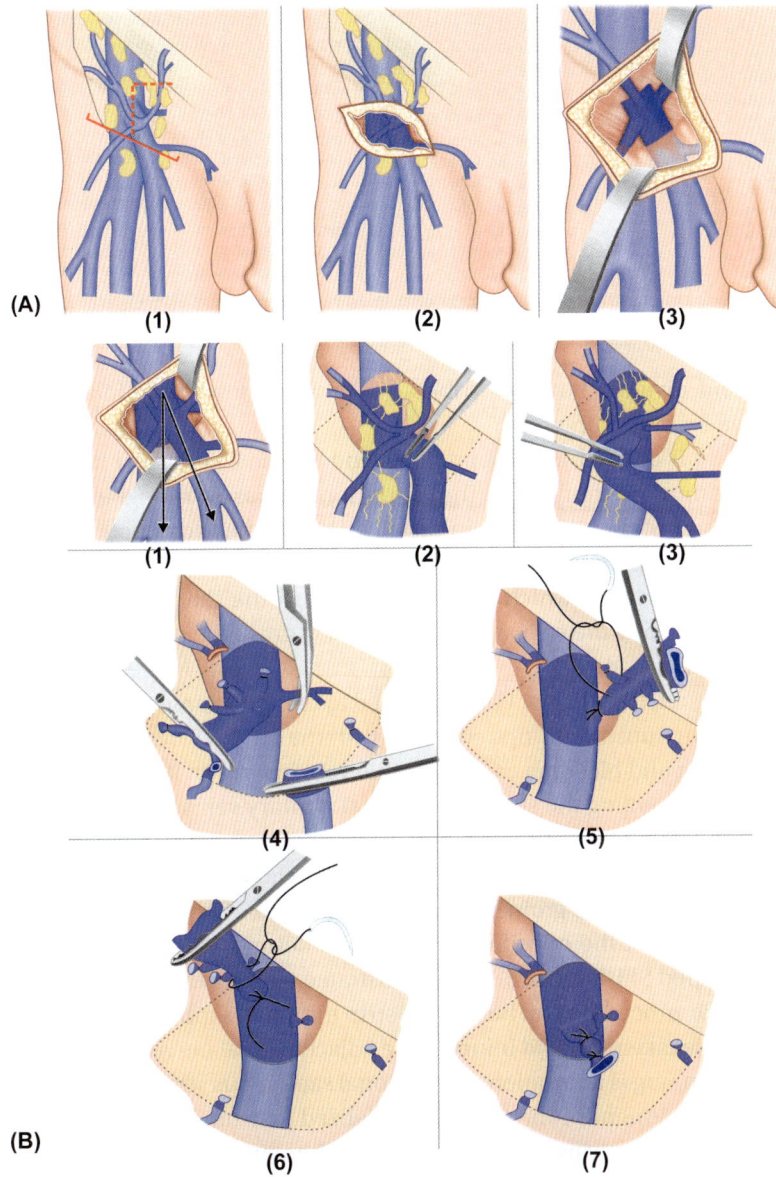

Figs. 11.3A and B: (A) Steps in the flush ligation of a long saphenous termination: (1) incision centered 2cm lateral to and below the pubic tubercle; (2) skin incision exposes the membranous layer of superficial fascia, which is incised separately; (3) fat is brushed downwards to expose the saphenous vein—the termination and its branches are cleared of fatty tissue. (B) Checking correct identity of saphenous vein: (1) it is not axial to the limb but inclines to the medial aspect—several typical branches are always present at the true termination; (2) and (3) the junction with the common femoral vein must be seen beyond doubt from both medial and lateral aspects; (4) once certain of its correct identity, the saphenous vein is divided and drawn forward to facilitate division of its branches; (5, 6 and 7) when fully isolated, the saphenous stump is ligated flush with the common femoral vein and then again, more peripherally, with a transfixion stitch.

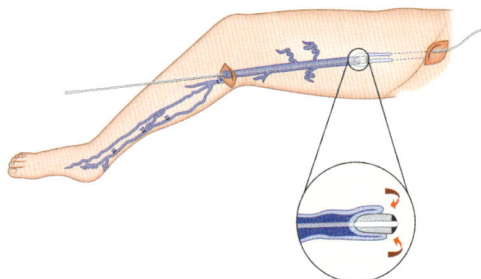

Fig. 11.4: Inversion stripping of the saphenous vein for superficial venous reflux caused by an incompetent saphenofemoral junction.

ligated and divided; however, tributaries draining the abdominal wall are preserved by some surgeons.

The GSV is divided, and the proximal end is flush ligated near its junction with the common femoral vein. The vein stripper is passed retrograde through the open end of the divided vein distally. Due to the incompetence of the vein valves, the stripper should pass easily. A small skin incision is made over the tip of the stripper, which is palpated through the skin, usually near the knee. After incising the vein, a forceps is used to grasp the stripper and pull it through the incision.

In the groin, the stripper is securely tied to the vein. Some surgeons prefer not to use the mushroom tips supplied with the stripper because excessive tissue trauma and bleeding can result. The vein inverts on itself and the vein is removed by pulling the stripper distally. Tributary veins that are tethering the vein can be disrupted using a percussion strike on the skin with four fingers as the stripper advances. Once hemostasis is achieved by direct pressure along the vein bed, the groin incision is closed with interrupted, absorbable suture. Closure of the cribriform fascia, with sutures or synthetic patches, over the ligated SFJ, has not been demonstrated to reduce groin recurrence.

A similar procedure can be used to strip the small saphenous vein (SSV). Care must be taken to avoid injury to the adjacent sural nerve.

Cryostripping is a variation of traditional saphenous stripping and is limited to the treatment of the GSV. A specialized instrument is placed at the level of the previously ligated and divided saphenous vein, and supercooled. The vein freezes adhering to the device and is removed as the device is pulled out. The reported advantage of this method is potentially reduced postoperative bruising compared with conventional techniques.[5]

SAPHENOPOPLITEAL JUNCTION LIGATION AND LESSER SAPHENOUS STRIPPING

Preoperative duplex to mark the position of the saphenopopliteal junction (SPJ) is highly recommended. The patient is positioned in the prone position, a transverse incision is made over the premarked SPJ, the fascia is divided and the SSV is exposed. The SPJ can then be formally dissected with a flush ligation or the SSV can be gently retracted and ligated as proximally as possible. No good evidence exists to favor one technique over the other, but proponents of the flush ligation would argue that it avoids leaving a stump of SSV, a common source of recurrence, while proponents of the simple SSV ligation technique argue that it reduces the incidence of the most common serious complications, nerve injury and popliteal vein injury. The SSV can then either be stripped or the proximal section of the vein can be resected. Those who strip, argue that it reduces the incidence of recurrence while opponents feel that it increases the incidence of sural nerve injury. There are no randomized trials comparing these techniques.

PERFORATOR LIGATION (FIGS. 11.5A AND B)

The majority of studies assessing the role of perforator ligation have been in patients with venous ulcers analyzing the effects on ulcer healing, and even in this situation randomized controlled data are lacking. The role of perforator ligation in patients with uncomplicated varicose veins is even less clear.

Open surgical subfascial perforator ligation (Linton procedure) was abandoned due to the magnitude of the operation and location of incisions in vulnerable areas of skin. The surgical site was prone to secondary ulceration when perforator ligation was not successful at reducing pressures within the skin. A much simple, open extrafascial perforator ligation can be performed via small incisions along Langer lines directly over the preoperatively marked blow-outs (incompetent perforators). The perforator forms a T-junction with

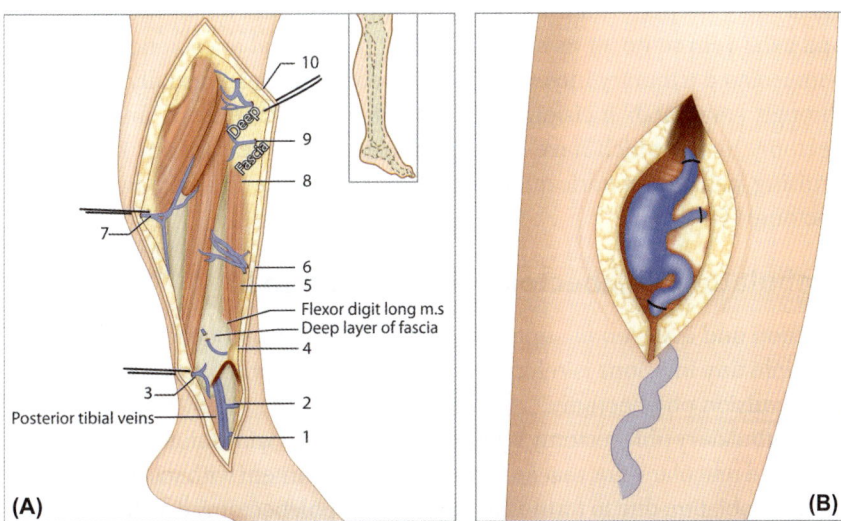

Figs. 11.5A and B: Picture showing perforator ligation at 3 sites.

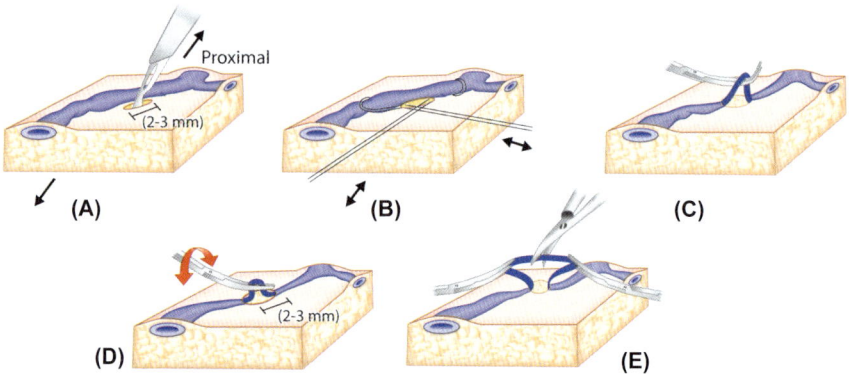

Figs. 11.6A to E: Technique of ambulatory phlebectomy (otherwise known as stab avulsions of varicosities.

the superficial vein, and above the T-junction, the vein is distended to form that which we refer as a 'blow-out'. Resection of the three veins forming the T-junction after careful individual ligation, and if necessary, a suture to the hole in deep fascia is all that is required. A less invasive surgical technique popularized in the 1980s used a videoscope placed through a small incision remote from the area of skin ulceration to identify and ligate perforating veins under direct vision. This technique, subfascial endoscopic perforator surgery, was used to treat patients with refractory symptoms or ulceration, or recurrent ulceration associated with perforator reflux.[6] However, this technique has also been largely abandoned in favor of minimally invasive techniques.

PHLEBECTOMIES

These may be performed following treatment of junctional incompetence and axial vein reflux or as sole treatment under local anesthetic in patients with isolated tributary incompetence. Phlebectomies are usually performed through small stab incisions using small mosquito forceps and/or phlebectomy hooks which have been demonstrated to be superior in terms of bruising, pain and generic quality of life than transilluminated powered phlebectomy (TIPP).

Ambulatory Phlebectomy (Figs. 11.6A to E)

Excision and avulsion of superficial varicosities (i.e., phlebectomy) through multiple tiny incisions is referred to as 'ambulatory phlebectomy' or 'microstab avulsion phlebectomy.'

Ambulatory phlebectomy is useful for removing a wide range of non-saphenous and reticular veins that are unsuitable for treatment with sclerotherapy, or catheter ablation due to tortuosity. Ambulatory phlebectomy can be combined with saphenous inversion for complete treatment at a single session.

We use an 18 gauge needle to make a series of punctures at intervals of 2–3 cm adjacent to the course of the marked veins. Sequential venous segments are engaged with a variety of small, specially designed crochet-like hooks, and are grasped and ligated or avulsed. Bleeding is controlled with direct pressure and limb elevation.

Transilluminated Powered Phlebectomy

Another technique for vein removal relies on the use of a powered, mechanical aspirator called TIPP. The device is similar to devices used by orthopedic surgeons to shave off cartilage. The device consists of a long, narrow tube that has a rotating blade at its tip to macerate and aspirate the target vein. An illuminator (light source) is placed into the subcutaneous tissue through a counterincision to improve visualization of the target veins through the skin.[7]

Following the administration of tumescent anesthesia, which is a mixture of saline, lidocaine and epinephrine, the device is inserted adjacent the path of the target vein. The blade is activated and the vein is aspirated into the device and destroyed.

The advantage of powered phlebectomy is the need for fewer incisions; however, systematic reviews have found that TIPP is associated with more postoperative pain and hematoma formation compared with ambulatory phlebectomy.[8,9] Another disadvantage of TIPP is the additional cost of the specialized equipment and supplies. Many patients with varicose veins also require management of saphenous reflux, which is often performed with an endovenous procedure. The combined equipment cost (i.e., endovenous plus TIPP) may be prohibitive, especially since cosmetic outcomes with TIPP do not appear superior to the conventional ligation/excision techniques described above.[9]

CONSERVATIVE VENOUS LIGATION

Conservative venous ligation (CHIVA; Conservatrice et Hémodynamique de l'Insuffisance Veineuse en Ambulatoire) is an alternative method that aims to disrupt the column of hydrostatic pressure by disconnecting points of venous reflux while preserving venous drainage.[10,11] The SFJ or SPJ is ligated and divided but not excised (i.e., stripped). Additional sites for ligation are identified with duplex ultrasound and clinical examination. A randomized trial of 501 patients found significantly lower visible vein recurrence rates at 5 years follow-up (intention-to-treat analysis) for patients managed with CHIVA compared with vein ligation/excision with exam-guided vein marking or vein ligation/excision with duplex-guided vein marking (40.1 versus 68.3 and 61.1% respectively).[12]

POSTOPERATIVE INSTRUCTIONS

Mild to moderate postoperative pain is common. Depending upon the extent of the vein excision, patients can be managed with extra strength acetaminophen or acetaminophen with codeine. Nonsteroidal anti-inflammatory agents may be added in patients who develop a significant phlebitic reaction.

Patients are encouraged to ambulate following surgery. The patient should make an effort to walk for 5-10 minutes each hour during waking hours. The patient should avoid prolonged standing and sitting. When not walking, the patient is encouraged to elevate the leg above the level of the heart.

Bruising along the tract of excised veins is common, and can take up to six weeks following surgery to resolve. Postoperative compression may help to limit bruising.

The operative dressings including the elastic bandages/stockings are maintained for several days. Once the operative dressing is removed, elastic stockings are worn during the day and removed at night.

Normal activities can be resumed when tolerated, usually within three to four days. Time off work varies between one and three weeks depending upon the patient's job requirements and the magnitude of the operation.

COMPLICATIONS OF STANDARD VARICOSE VEIN SURGERY

Complications (minor and major) are reported in up to 20% of patients who undergo traditional varicose vein surgery. Wound infections, the most common complication, are reduced by prophylactic antibiotics. Nerve injury is the most common serious complication. The incidence of saphenous nerve neuralgia is up to 7% following long saphenous vein stripping to the knee (the incidence is higher with stripping to the ankle). The incidence of sural nerve neuropraxia and common peroneal nerve injury may be as high as 20 and 4% respectively following SSV surgery. The incidence of venous thromboembolic complications is approximately 0.5% following varicose vein surgery; however, patient risk factors must be individually assessed and appropriate prophylaxis administered according to guidelines.

MINIMAL INVASIVE METHODS

After the axial venous incompetence is addressed and treated. Secondary branch varicosities are also addressed. Finally, treatment options for spider veins are considered. These include injection sclerotherapy, laser treatment and radioablation.

Injection Sclerotherapy

The venectasia can be ablated successfully using the injection sclerotherapy technique. Dilute solutions of sclerosant (e.g., 1–3% sodium sotradecol solution) can be injected directly into the venules. Care must be taken to ensure that no single injection dose exceeds 0.1 mL but that multiple injections completely fill all feeding vessels. When the session is complete, a pressure dressing is applied, consisting of cotton balls at each injection site, and then covered with a pressure dressing of Coban wrap or low-grade compression stockings. Patients are advised to ambulate frequently over the first 24 hours, to abstain from direct sun exposure and airline travel for 2 weeks. Occasionally, entrapped blood may form, and patients report significant discomfort. Needle drainage is performed at the site, which facilitates healing and cosmesis, and rapidly improves discomfort. This liberation of entrapped blood is as important to success as the primary injection. This therapy is remarkably successful in achieving an excellent cosmetic result. In patients with a known allergy to sodium tetradecyl (Sotradecol), hypertonic saline can be used. Pain can occur with the use of pure hypertonic solutions, so lidocaine is added to the solution to decrease discomfort. Venules larger than 1 mm and smaller than 3 mm can also be injected with a sclerosant of slightly greater concentration, but the amount injected needs to be limited to less than 0.5 mL. Although injection sclerotherapy has met with significant success, complications do occur. They include hyperpigmentation, venous matting, postsclerotherapy necrosis and an allergic reaction to the sclerosant. In addition, telangiectasia formation after injection sclerotherapy treatment tends to recur. Patients will commonly observe return of spider veins from 8 to 12 months after treatment. Although patients may report localized discomfort, sclerotherapy of telangiectasias is considered cosmetic and does not influence the venous circulation of the extremity.

Foam Sclerotherapy

Foam sclerotherapy is a modality that has been introduced in Europe and has achieved great success, not only with spider veins, but also as a treatment option for perforator vein ablation. However, paradoxical embolism can occur, which is the main reason that foam sclerosant therapy has not been widely used in the United States. Standardization of technique and formal studies will likely demonstrate the appropriate safety of foam sclerotherapy for venous therapy.

Laser Treatment

Laser treatment of spider telangiectasias has been performed using a variety of wavelengths and varying techniques, such as high intensity pulsed light, fiber guided laser coagulation and Nd:YAG laser with a wavelength of

1,064 nm. Evaluation of all existing laser modalities has suggested that the Nd:YAG laser has the most success. However, to date, there have not been any prospective randomized trials to support this presumption. Laser treatment does tend to be more painful. Laser treatment in most centers will be used in conjunction with injection sclerotherapy—that is, injection treats the feeding venules; laser treatment will be used to treat the extremely small branches not adequately addressed with the injection technique. Most patients are satisfied with the injection only method.

RADIOFREQUENCY ABLATION

Radiofrequency (RF) thermal energy is delivered directly to the vessel wall, causing protein denaturation, collagenous contraction and immediate closure of the vessel. In contrast to laser therapy, the RF catheter actually comes into contact with the lumen walls.

An introducer sheath is inserted into the proposed vein of treatment (again usually the GSV). A special RF ablation catheter is passed through the sheath and along the vein until the active tip is at the SFJ just distal to the subterminal valve. Just like the endovenous laser, tumescent local anesthetic is injected.

Metal fingers at the tip of the RF catheter are deployed until they make contact with the vessel endothelium. RF energy is delivered, both in and around the vessel to be treated. Thermal sensors record the temperature within the vessel and deliver just enough energy to ensure endothelial ablation. The RF catheter is withdrawn a short distance, and the process is repeated all along the length of the vein to be treated.

RECURRENT VARICOSE VEINS

Approximately 10–20% of patients who present to hospital with varicose veins have had previous intervention. Prospective data on long-term results following intervention for recurrent varicose veins are sparse and the criteria for defining recurrence are variable.

Significant clinical recurrence five to ten years following varicose vein surgery occurs in 10–35% of patients, but minor/duplex detected recurrence is much more common being in the order of 70%. Causes of recurrence are controversial but include: neo-revascularization, reflux in residual axial vein, inadequate initial surgery and new junctional reflux. Recurrence is more common following short than long saphenous vein surgery and in patients with high BMI (body mass index), while stripping of the incompetent axial vein reduces recurrence rates. Limited data suggest recurrence rates following endovenous thermal ablation may be lower and of different etiology (axial vein recanalization) than following surgery. Recurrent varicose veins often have an atypical distribution and duplex assessment is mandatory. Surgery for recurrent varicose veins is associated with a high (40%) complication rate, the most common being lymph leak and wound infection, thus endovenous interventions would b to offer an attractive alternative, where feasible.

COMPARISON OF INTERVENTIONS

Endovenous and traditional surgery for varicose veins appear equally beneficial in improving generic and disease-specific quality of life in the short to medium term. However, in the early postoperative period, traditional surgery is associated with higher pain scores and analgesic requirement, and more severe disability in terms of physical, social and psychological quality of life although the clinical significance of this is unclear. Thus, endovenous interventions, by minimizing the immediate postoperative quality of life impairment, result in a more rapid return to work and normal activities. Adequately powered, long-term comparisons of recurrence rates following surgery and endovenous interventions are awaited.

REFERENCES

1. Williams NS, Bulstrode CJK, O'Connell PR. Bailey & Love's Short Practice of Surgery (26th edition). London: Hodder Arnold; 2013.
2. Townsend C, Beauchamp RD, Evers BM, et al. Sabiston Textbook of Surgery: the Biological Basis of Modern Surgical Practice (19th and 20th edition). Philadelphia: Elsevier Inc; 2016.
3. Morris PJ, Wood WC. Oxford Textbook of Surgery (2nd edition). London: Oxford University Press; 2000.
4. Foote RR. Varicose Veins: A Practical Manual; R Rowden Foote (3rd edition). Bristol: John Wright & Sons Limited; 1960.
5. Menyhei G, Gyevnár Z, Arató E, et al. Conventional stripping versus cryostripping: a prospective randomised trial to compare improvement in quality of life and complications. Eur J Vasc Endovasc Surg. 2008;35(2):218-23.
6. Gloviczki P, Bergan JJ, Menawat SS, et al. Safety, feasibility, and early efficacy of subfascial endoscopic perforator surgery: a preliminary report from the North American registry. J Vasc Surg. 1997;25(1):94-105.
7. Crane J, Cheshire N. Recent developments in vascular surgery. BMJ. 2003; 327(7420):911-5.
8. Luebke T, Brunkwall J. Meta-analysis of transilluminated powered phlebectomy for superficial varicosities. J Cardiovasc Surg (Torino). 2008;49(6):757-64.
9. Scavée V. Transilluminated powered phlebectomy: not enough advantages? Review of the literature. Eur J Vasc Endovasc Surg. 2006;31(3):316-9.
10. Franceschi C. Théorie et practique de la cure conservatrice et hémodynamique de l'insuffisance veineuse en ambulatoire. Précyy-sous-thil, France: Edition de l'Aramançon, 1988.
11. Criado, E, Juan J, Fontcuberta J, et al. Haemodynamic surgery for varicose veins: rationale, and anatomic and haemodynamic basis. Phlebology. 2003;18(4):158-66.
12. Parés JO, Juan J, Tellez R, et al. Varicose vein surgery: stripping versus the CHIVA method: a randomized controlled trial. Ann Surg. 2010;251(4):624-31.

Index

Note: Page numbers followed by *f* refer to figure and *t* refer to table.

A

Alcohol intoxication 55
Allergic reactions 86, 94
Ambulatory phlebectomy, technique of 116*f*
Ambulatory venous pressure 36
  interpretation of 38*t*
Anaphylaxis 86
Ankle
  flare 21
  joint stiffness 26
  perforators 8
  venous flare 19
Arterial occlusive disease, advanced peripheral 65
Arteriovenous fistula 94
Artery hypertension, pulmonary 55
Aspiration 102, 104
Asthma, bronchial 65
Atrophie blanche 19, 24
Automated foaming device turbofoam 96

B

Bassi's perforator 9
Bedside tests 31
  validation of 34
Bicuspid valves 5
Bleomycin 47, 56
Blood coagulum, manual extraction of 95*f*
Blue veins 16
Body mass index 120
Brodie-Trendelenburg test 32
  demonstration of 32*f*
  interpretation of 33*t*
Bronchospasm 55

C

Cabrera's technique 75
Calf muscles 7
Calf perforators, lateral 9
Carbon dioxide 76
  laser 104, 106
Cerebrovascular accidents 90
Chemical
  irritants 54
  phlebitis post-sclerotherapy 88
Chromated glycerin 47, 54, 60
Cockett's perforators 3
Compression
  after sclerotherapy, types of 43
  bandage 42
    application of 44
  elastic 42
  elastocrepe for 66
  hosiery 42
  therapy 41
  types of 42
Compressive therapy, mechanism of action of 41
Computed tomography 34, 38
Concertina method 111
Contact dermatitis 22, 98
  allergic 86
Corona phlebectatica paraplantaris 21
Cough impulse test 31
Cramps 19
Cryosurgery 102, 104
Cystic
  hygroma 105
  lesions 100
Cysts
  epidermoid 100
  ganglion 48

mucous 101, 102
oral mucous 100

D

Deep plantar arch 6
Deep vein thrombosis 64, 91
　history of 65
Dermatitis 64
Detergent sclerosant 77
Diathesis, allergic 65
Disrupt vein cellular membrane 47
Distended varicose veins, persistence of 34
Dodd's and Hunterian perforators 9
Doppler ultrasonography 35, 37f, 38
Doppler ultrasound machine 36f
Dorsalis pedis 6
Duplex ultrasonography 35

E

Eczema 22
　acute 23f
　chronic 23f
Edema 20, 30, 87, 94
Embolia cutis medicamentosa 93
Embolism, pulmonary 91, 92
Endosclerosis 46
Endothelial
　activation 17
　cell 46
　damage 46
Endothelium, direct caustic destruction
　　of 47
Epinephrine 95f
Erysipelas 24
Ethanol 47, 55
　deep penetration 55
Ethanolamine oleate 47, 50, 60
Excision 104
Extracellular matrix 17f
　degradation 17

F

Fascia lata 31f
Fascial compartments of leg, superficial 1f
Fegan's technique 68, 69
Femoral vein 2
Femur, adductor tubercle of 2

Fibrin cuff theory 25
Fixed plantar flexion 27
Foam
　preparation 78f
　　methods of 75
　sclerotherapy 44, 75, 82, 86, 89, 119
　　advantages of 82
　　peroperative 75
　stability 76
　types of 77
Foot
　perforators 8, 9
　veins of 2f
Fossa ovalis 31f

G

Gallbladder ablation 48
Gastrointestinal bleeding, upper 48
Glycerin 58, 95f
Graduated compression stockings 43

H

Hemangiomas 100
Hematoma 111
Hemoglobinuria 55, 94
Hemorrhage 21
Hyperpigmentation 15, 96
　post-sclerotherapy 90f, 96
Hypersensitivity reactions 86
Hyperthermia 55
Hyperthyroidism 65
Hypertonic
　saline 51, 53, 58, 71, 86
　sodium chloride solution 47, 59
Hypoallergenic tape 66

I

Ideal compression system, properties of 41
Infection 93, 97
Ischemic attack, transient 90
Itching 19

K

Kaposi sarcoma 48
Keller method 111
Klippel-Trenaunay syndrome 16
Knee perforators 8

L

Laplace's law 77
Laser
  ablation 102
  treatment 119
Leg
  edema 65
  perforator 8
  ulcers, proximity of 86
Leonardo's vein 2
Lidocaine 58, 95f
Linear bullae from tape 88f
Linton procedure 111, 115
Lipodermatosclerosis 15, 19, 23, 24f, 27, 30f
Liquid sclerotherapy 44, 86, 89
Lobular capillary hemangioma 106
Lower leg, ulceration of 26
Lower limb
  deep veins of 6f
  major perforator veins of 10f
  perforators of 14f
  pigmentation of 22f
Lymphangioma 100, 104
  cavernous 105
  circumscriptum 104, 105, 107f
Lymphedema 27, 87, 94
Lymphoceles 48

M

Magnetic resonance imaging 34, 39, 105
Matrix metalloproteinases 17
Medial calf perforators 9
Metalloproteinase, tissue inhibitor of 17f
Micro-marsupialization technique 102
Microsclerotherapy 71
Micro-stab avulsion phlebectomy 116
Microvascular valves 10
Migraine 65, 90
Minimal invasive methods 118
Minocycline 89
Montreux technique 76, 77
Mucocele 102f, 103f
Multi-layer bandaging systems 42
Muscle cramps 30

N

Necrosis 92, 97
Neovascularization 89f

Nerve
  impairment 55
  injury 90
Nonsteroidal anti-inflammatory drugs 96

O

Ok 432 47, 56
Oliguria, transient 94
Oral lesions, percutaneous ablation of 48
Oral ranulas, treatment of 102
Orbach's air block 77
Osmotic solutions 51

P

Pain 30, 27, 64
Paresthesia 19
Patent foramen ovale 90
Pelvic
  origin, varicose veins of 86
  vascular lesion 39f
Percussion test 31
Perforating veins, incompetent 64, 86
Perforators
  ligation 115, 115f
  nomenclature 8t
  old and new terminologies of 14t
  paratibial 9
  thigh 8, 9
Periostitis 27
Peripheral arterial occlusive disease 65
Peripheral calf muscle pump 7f
Perthes test 33, 34
  demonstration of 33f
  interpretation of 34t
  modified 33
Phlebectomy 116
  ambulatory 116
Phlebitis, superficial 19
Pigmentation 22, 89, 94
  post-sclerotherapy 89
Plethysmography 38
Polidocanol 47, 49, 58, 59, 68, 75, 85, 87f, 88f, 101
Polyethylene-oxide chain 49
Polyiodinated iodine 47, 55, 60
Pressure erythema 22
Protein theft denaturation 47
Pruritus 30
Pubic tubercle 31f, 113f
Pyogenic granuloma 100, 106, 108f

Q

Q-switched laser 96

R

Radiofrequency
    ablation 120
    thermal energy 120
Ranula 101, 102, 103*f*
Restless legs 19
Reticular veins 15, 16, 21*f*, 58, 69
Rindfleisch-Friedel procedure 111

S

Salivary gland 101
Saphenofemoral junction 2, 3, 4*f*, 93, 111
    incompetence 65, 114*f*
Saphenofemoral ligation 112
Saphenopopliteal junction 4, 5*f*, 93, 114
    ligation 114
Saphenous nerve 10
Saphenous stripping
    lesser 114
    long 112
Saphenous vein
    greater 2, 3*f*, 13, 31, 31*f*, 64, 111
    incompetent 64, 86
    inversion stripping of 114*f*
    lesser 31, 64
    short 13
    small 2, 4, 5*f*, 91, 114
    superficial 87
Scarring 15
Sclerosant 46, 65
    concentration of 67, 68*t*
Sclerosing agents 47*t*, 58, 58*t*-60*t*, 78
Sclerosing solutions 46, 65, 66
Sclerotherapy 41, 43, 63-65, 69, 71, 71*f*, 73, 80, 85, 100, 102, 104, 105*f*, 106, 107, 108*f*, 119
    complications of 85
    contraindications of 86*t*
    indications of 64, 86*t*
    mechanism of 63
    objectives of 63
    over surgical procedures 108
    procedure 100
    purpose of 46
    techniques 68
    tray 67*f*
Sebaceous cyst 100, 101*f*
Sigg's technique 68, 69
Skin
    irritation 30, 87, 97
    necrosis 55, 93*f*
    pigmentation 30
Smooth muscle
    apoptosis dysregulation 17
    cell 17, 17*f*
Sodium
    chloride solution with dextrose 47, 58, 60
    morrhuate 47, 50, 59
    sotradecol solution 119
    tetradecyl sulfate 47, 48, 58, 59, 68, 69, 85, 101, 103*f*
Spider veins 16, 86
Standard varicose vein surgery, complications of 118
Static stiffness index 42
Steatocystoma multiplex 104, 104*f*
Stroke 90
Subdermic venous system, lateral 13
Superficial
    compartment of venous system of leg, anatomy of 13*f*
    fascia, layer of 113*f*
    vein thrombosis, acute 64
Sural nerve 10
Swelling 19
Systemic disease, severe 65

T

Tap test 31
Telangiectasia 15, 16, 20, 58, 71, 86, 95*f*
    microsclerotherapy of 71
Tessari method 75, 76*f*
Thrombophilia 65
Thrombophlebitis, superficial 21, 87
Thrombosis, superficial 91
Thrombus formation 92*f*
Tissue plasminogen activator 25
Topical nitroglycerine ointment 66
Total endothelial destruction 47
Transilluminated powered phlebectomy 116, 117
Trendelenburg test 34
    modified 32
Tumors, hemorrhagic 48

U

Ulcer 15, 24, 27, 30
  healing 30f
  varicose 23f, 27f
Ultrasound guided sclerotherapy 72, 72f, 85
  techniques of 72
Urticaria 86
  post-injection 87f

V

Valsalva maneuvers 98
Valves 5
  dysfunction 16
Variceal bleeding 48
Varices 16
Varicoceles 48
Varicose veins 15-17, 19, 20f, 30f, 34, 39f, 41, 57, 63, 64, 86
  ablation of 64
  complications of 64
  emptying of 34
  evaluation of 29
  formation 17f
  large 58
  pathophysiology of 13
  presentation 19t
  recurrent 120
  residual and recurrent 64, 86
  reticular 64, 86
  sclerotherapy, principles of 67
  surgical treatment of 111
Vascular
  fibrosis 64
  malformation 48, 58
  obliteration 64
Veins
  diameter 80
  examination of 36f
  length 80
  perforating 7, 8, 13
  refluxing 86
  superficial 1, 2, 5, 111
  thread 16
  X-ray of 35f
Venogram 35f
Venography 34, 35
Venous
  anatomy 1
  dilatation 16
  diseases 13
  disorders
    chronic 64
    of lower limb 1
  eczema 19
  hypertension 13
  insufficiency 19
    chronic 15, 16, 29, 38, 63
    primary 15
    symptoms suggestive of 29, 30
  ligation, conservative 117
  malformations 86
  pathophysiology 15
  physiology 15f
  pressure 14, 42
  reflux, superficial 114f
  sinuses 7
  system
    of lower limbs 13, 14
    superficial 72
    varicosities, lateral 64
  telangiectasia 19
  thrombosis, superficial 24, 92
  ulceration, mechanism of 25
  ulcers 19, 22, 26, 63, 64
Venule 58
Venulectasia 16
Visual disturbances 90

W

White blood cell 25
White cell trapping theory 25

X

X-ray of veins 35f